Khédija SOUMER
Adel MRAD

Medium- and long-term results of valve bioprostheses

Khédija SOUMER
Adel MRAD

Medium- and long-term results of valve bioprostheses

Tunisian multicentre study

ScienciaScripts

Contents

To *our Master and President of the jury*
Professor Amine JEMEL
Head of the Department of Cardiovascular Surgery
CHU Abderrahmen Mami
*You have done us the great honour of accepting to chair our
thesis jury.*
*We have the deep and abiding respect for you that comes from your
innumerable human and professional qualities.*
*Your kindness, competence, rigour in your work and the
high quality of your teaching have always aroused our admiration
and gratitude.*
*We shall remain devoted to your principles and faithful to your precious advice
. Please accept, dear master, the*
sincere
expression of
*our deepest gratitude and consideration for
this work.*
To our Master and Judge
Professor Feker GHEDIRA
Department of Cardiovascular Surgery
CHU La Rabta
*We are very touched by the honour you have done us by agreeing to
judge this thesis.*
*Your outstanding human qualities, your unfailing pedagogical spirit and
your immaculate rigour are a noble ideal for us.*
*Your generosity and your advice will always mark us
Please find in this work the expression of our great admiration
and our deep gratitude.*
To our Master and Judge
Professor Agrege Emna BENNOUR
Cardiology Department
CHU Abderrahmen Mami
*It is a great honour to have you on our
esteemed panel of judges.*
*We have the utmost
respect and admiration for your human and professional qualities*
.
*Please find in this work the expression of our
most sincere gratitude*
To *our Master and Judge*
Professor Agrege Mokhles LAJMI

Department of Cardiovascular and Thoracic Surgery
Hôpital militaireprincipal'dinstructwn de Tunis
We are very honoured that you have agreed to sit on
our jury.
Your human and professional qualities are bound to inspire esteem and
respect.
Your kindness, your attentiveness and your invaluable advice will never
be forgotten.
May this work be a token of our
deepest and most sincere gratitude

To our Master and Judge
Professor Agrege Mouna BOUSNINA
Department of Cardiovascular Surgery
CHU Abderrahmen Mami
We thank you for the honour of being on
our jury and for the attention you have paid to this work.
We have the utmost respect for your competence and availability.
Please find in this work the expression of our
sincerest thanks

To our Master and Rapporteur of these
Professor Mohamed ZIADI
Department of Cardiovascular and Thoracic Surgery
Hôpital militaireprincipal d'instruction de Tunis
You have done us a great honour by agreeing to report on this work.
We have always
admired your kindness, generosity and knowledge.
Your availability, your advice and your invaluable comments were
an unquestionable help in carrying out this work.
Please accept our deepest gratitude and
respect.

Dr Khedija SOUMER
Department of Cardiovascular Surgery
CHU Abderrahmen Mami
I am touched by the honour you have done me by agreeing to
direct me
in this work.
I would like to thank you for your availability, your attentiveness and your
enlightened advice
along the way.
Without your guidance and patience, this work would never have seen the
light of day.

*Please accept the expression of my deepest gratitude and
consideration.*
***To our Master and guest of honour
Professor Raouf DENGUIR
Head of Cardiovascular Surgery Department
CHU La Rabta***
*Thank you to you and to the entire team at La Rabta Cardiovascular Surgery
for accompanying and guiding me throughout my residency.
We have the utmost
respect and admiration for your human and professional qualities*

*Please find in this work the expression of our
most sincere gratitude.*

2 INTRODUCTION

Over 250,000 valve prostheses are implanted each year worldwide, and more than half of these are bioprostheses [1]. In developing countries, with very little access to cardiac surgery, the incidence of valve replacement is estimated at 4.75 per 100,000 population [2].

The first heart valve replacements were performed in the 1960s. Since then, valve surgery has continued to evolve, aiming to restore the function of the damaged valve, with three parallel, or even competing, options: conservative or reparative surgery, so-called "mechanical" prostheses and biological valves [3].

When a defective heart valve does not lend itself to conservative treatment, the surgeon is obliged to replace it with a prosthesis. In such a situation, the ideal would be to implant a prosthetic valve with the same hemodynamic performance as a native valve, with long durability and without the need for long-term anticoagulation. Such a prosthesis does not yet exist.

Mechanical prostheses, known for their excellent durability, require permanent curative anticoagulant treatment, which is associated with potentially serious risks of haemorrhage. Biological prostheses, on the other hand, are characterised by their good blood tolerance on contact and do not require anticoagulation, but have a more limited lifespan [3].

The choice of a cardiac prosthesis was based on two essential parameters: age and anticoagulant treatment. Patients over 65-70 will receive a bioprosthesis that does not require anticoagulation but is likely to deteriorate, while patients under 65 will be more likely to receive a mechanical prosthesis and will be subject to lifelong anticoagulation treatment.

This theory has been rectified over time, and the proportion of biological valves implanted has risen steadily to far exceed that of mechanical valves. In fact, over the last few decades, continuous innovation in bioprosthesis design, manufacture and preservation techniques over the last 30 years has improved both performance and durability, and has led to a change in the criteria for choosing the type of valve prosthesis, which is increasingly based on the wishes of the properly informed patient and his or her lifestyle [4].

In recent years, the rate of surgical implantation of bioprostheses has increased significantly. This rate has risen from 22.5% in 2006 to 76.8% in 2016, compared with a significant decrease in the rate of implantation of mechanical valves, from 77.5% in 2006 to 23.2% in 2016 [5].

With the new generation of bioprostheses, the hemodynamic characteristics of these substitutes, their longevity and the fact that there is no need for anticoagulant treatment with its haemorrhagic complications, biological prostheses have become the alternative of choice for patients of all ages.

In this work, we propose to present a series of patients who have undergone valve replacement(s) using a bioprosthesis at three cardiovascular surgery centres.

The objectives of our study were to:

- Analysing the clinical and evolutionary profile of patients who have undergone valve replacement with a biological prosthesis
- To study the factors predictive of post-operative morbidity and mortality.

3 METHODS

I. STUDY POPULATION :

This is a retrospective, multicentre, descriptive, cross-sectional study conducted in the cardiovascular surgery departments of the Abderrahman Mami University Hospital in Ariana, the Habib Bourguiba Hospital in Sfax, and the Main Military Training Hospital in Tunis, between September 2017 and December 2021.

1. Inclusion criteria :

We included in the study all patients who had one or more bioprostheses in any position (mitral, aortic and/or tricuspid), whether or not associated with coronary surgery.

2. Non-inclusion criteria :

Not included:

- Patients who have had valve replacement(s) using mechanical prosthesis(es)
- Patients who had undergone surgery on the ascending thoracic aorta. This last group was not included so as not to bias the predictive factors of post-operative morbidity and mortality.

3. Exclusion criteria :

Patients with medical records that could not be used due to a lack of observation notebooks, per-operative data or post-operative follow-up were excluded.

II. AIMS OF THE STUDY :

To describe the clinical and evolutionary profile of patients who have undergone valve replacement with a biological prosthesis and to study the factors predictive of post-operative morbidity and mortality.

III. CONDUCT OF THE STUDY :

Epidemiological and clinical data were collected from medical records according to a pre-established data processing form specifying several variables extracted from these records (Appendix 1). This included :

1. Epidemiological data :

Age at admission, gender, occupation, weight and height to determine body mass index (BMI), cardiovascular risk factors including diabetes, hypertension, smoking, dyslipidemia and Euroscore II were recorded.

The Euroscore II or European System for Cardiac Operative Risk Evaluation predicts mortality by calculating the probability of peri-operative death.

2. Factors related to the terrain :

We identified factors related to the patient's condition that could modify the peri-operative context. These factors were divided into three groups:

2.1. Medical history :

We have noted :

- The presence of other concomitant pathologies such as cerebrovascular accident, chronic bronchopneumopathy (COPD), chronic renal insufficiency (CRI), the association of coronary artery disease (CAD), etc., may be a factor in the development of the disease.
- The concept of addiction
- Taking anticoagulants or platelet anti-aggregants

In order to address the risks associated with the use of anticoagulants or platelet anti-aggregants, these were stopped before 3 days of the operation for oral anticoagulants and before 24 hours for anti-aggregants.

2.2. Factors related to valvulopathy :

We found :

-    History of rheumatic fever
-    History of percutaneous mitral dilatation
-    The context of infectious endocarditis
-    History of cardiac surgery such as mitral or aortic valve replacement or closed mitral commissurotomy

2.3. Factors that may aggravate the surgical procedure :

Factors that could influence the risk of the operation were taken into account, such as the emergency context and the time taken to perform the operation in relation to the diagnosis of the valve disease.

3. Preoperative assessment of patients :

3.1. Clinical data :

Patients were referred from cardiology departments and by free-lance cardiologists. They were seen on an outpatient basis or admitted in an emergency setting.

Each patient was assessed for functional impairment including dyspnoea according to the NYHA classification and other concomitant symptoms such as chest pain, syncope and equivalent, signs of right and/or left heart failure and embolic events.

3.2. Paraclinical data :

All patients had :

■   A pre-operative biological work-up, an electrocardiogram to look for rhythm and conduction disorders, whether or not associated with ischemic signs, and a frontal chest X-ray to determine the cardiothoracic ratio and analyse the cardiac silhouette.

■   A transthoracic Doppler echocardiogram showing the following:

■   Involvement of the mitral and/or aortic and/or tricuspid valves with quantification of the degree of stenosis or leakage

■   Left ventricular ejection fraction

■   Impact on the heart chambers, in particular left ventricular hypertrophy/dilatation and/or dilatation of the right chambers

■   Segmental kinetic disorders

■   Pulmonary arterial pressures

■   The presence of vegetation, abscesses or thrombi

Patients aged over 45 underwent pre-operative coronary angiography to identify associated coronary disease, and ultrasound of the supra-aortic trunks to look for possible carotid stenosis.

3.3. Anaesthetic evaluation :

All patients were seen and assessed by an anaesthetist prior to surgery.

4. Operating data :

4.1. Preparation and installation of the patient :

The operation was performed under general anaesthetic. Intra- and post-operative monitoring was based on measurement of blood pressure, heart rate, o_2 saturation, diuresis, core temperature, finger blood glucose, electrocardiogram, respiratory monitoring and biological monitoring with blood gas, blood ionogram, blood count and lactate assay.

The standard patient position is supine, with the legs together and the arms held at the sides of the body. The operator is positioned on the patient's right, with the assistant on the opposite side (Figure 1).

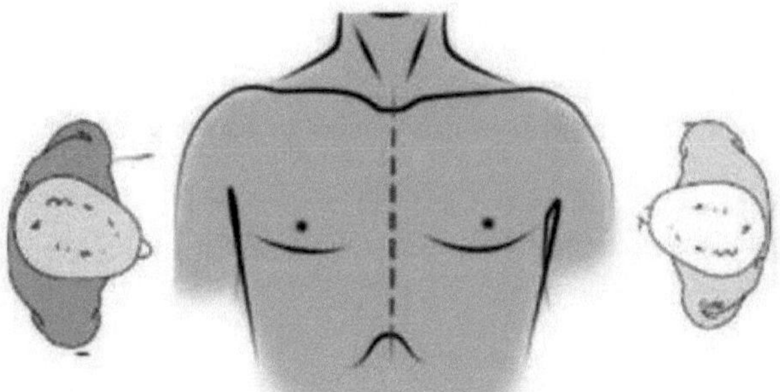

Figure 1: Patient positioning [6].

4.2.APPROACHES :
4.2.1. Median vertical sternotomy :
This is the classic approach in cardiac surgery. It consists of opening the sternum vertically through the middle, allowing exposure of the anterior mediastinum and access to the creur and large vessels (Figure 2). This allows rapid and easy installation of the bypass graft and valve replacement under optimum conditions.
4.2.2. Mini-sternotomy :
It consists of a small midline incision followed by opening of the upper half of the sternal bone (Figure 2).

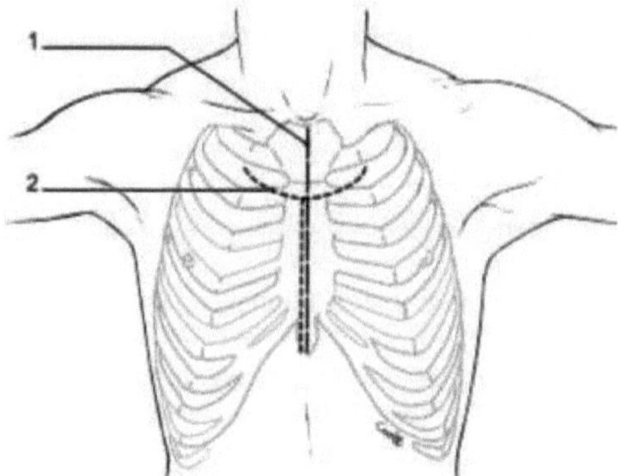

Figure 2: Cutaneous incisions of the sternum using different approaches [6].
1. Median vertical sternotomy
2. Mini-sternotomy

4.3.PROCEEDINGS OF THE CEC :
All valve replacements have been carried out under CEC, the only way of obtaining an exsanguinated and immobile heart, which are essential conditions for resection of the valve and fitting of the cardiac prosthesis.

After opening the pericardium and obtaining effective anticoagulation with 3 mg/kg sodium heparin, we proceeded to place the bypass graft between the aorta and the right atrium.

Aortic cannulation takes place at the foot of the brachiocephalic arterial trunk. Venous cannulation was single in the case of isolated aortic valve replacement and double via the superior and inferior vena cava in the case of mitral and/or tricuspid valve replacement.

Lakes were placed around the vena cava in the event of a procedure on the tricuspid to completely isolate the heart muscle from the bloodstream and prevent pump failure. The heart muscle was stopped by injecting a cardioplegia solution at the time of aortic clamping. This was passed through the root of the aorta, or selectively via the coronary ostia in the case of aortic valve replacement, allowing the heart to be stopped while preserving the integrity of the organ.

4.4. ROUTE OF EXPOSURE OF THE VALVE :

4.4.1. Left auriculotomy:

The mitral valve was approached via a left atriotomy allowing good exposure of the valve. The incision was made behind Sondergaard's sulcus, in line with the right superior pulmonary vein. The incision is then extended in an arcuate fashion under the inferior vena cava (Figure 3).

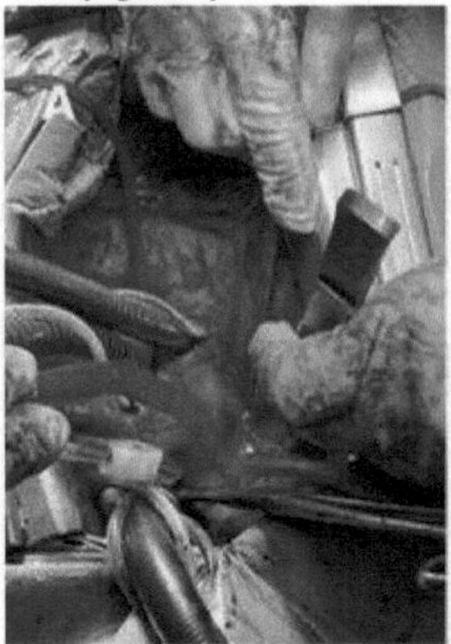
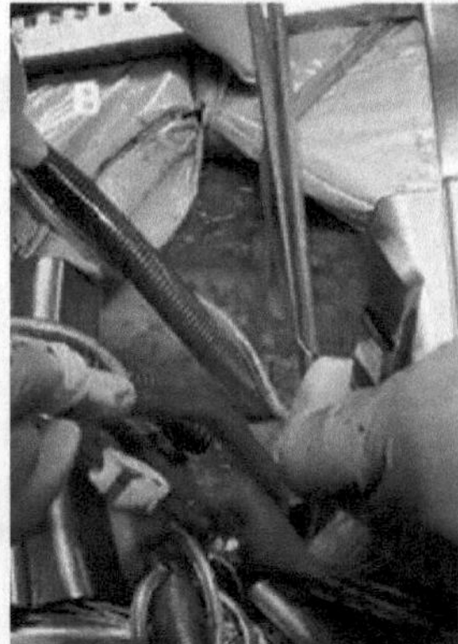
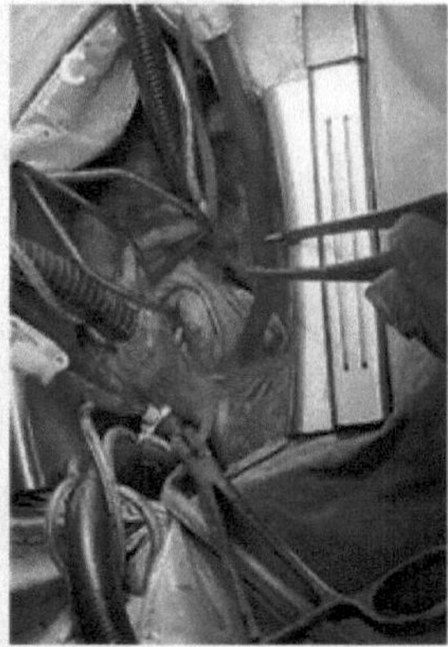

Figure 3: Left auriculotomy
A- Initiation of the left atrial incision opposite Sondergaard's groove.
8- Enlargement of the incision over the right superior pulmonary vein. C- Left atrium opened via a left atriotomy exposing the mitral valve.

4.4.2. Right auriculotomy:

We gained access to the tricuspid valve through a right atriotomy, incising parallel to the right atrioventricular groove and extending from the atrium towards the inferior vena cava (Figure 4).

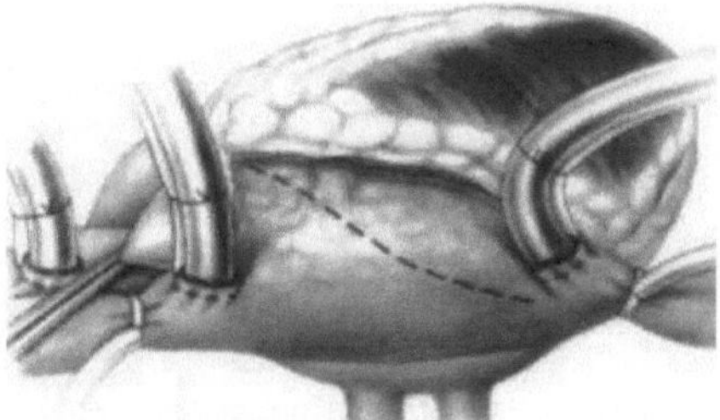

Figure 4: Oblique right auriculotomy [7].

4.4.3. Trans-aortic route :

To approach the aortic valve, we performed a transverse or oblique aortotomy on the anterior surface of the aorta. The incision was extended upwards towards the pulmonary artery, obliquely downwards towards the middle of the non-coronary sinus, stopping one cm from the annulus (Figure 5).

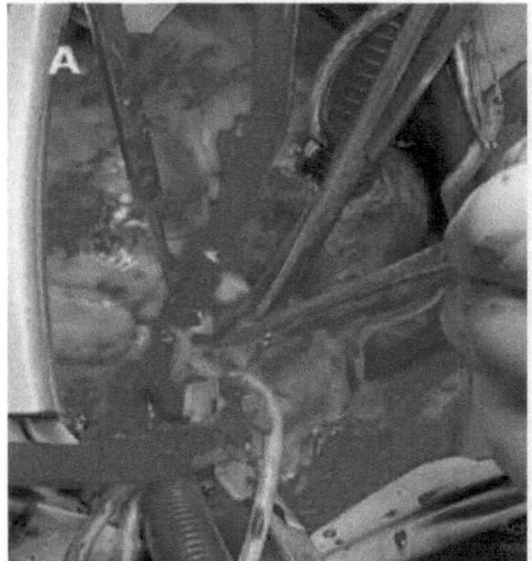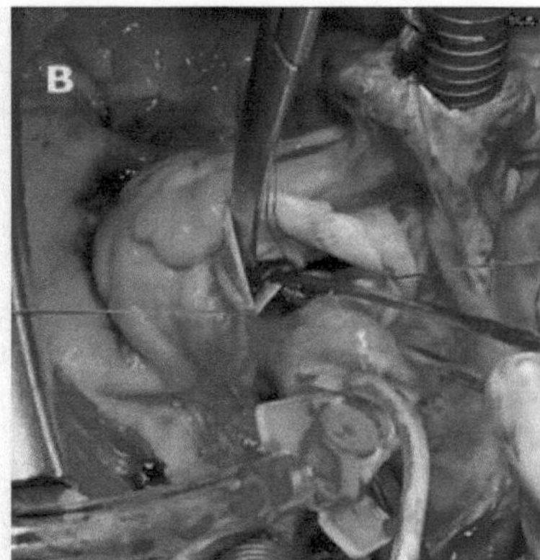

Figure 5: Surgical view of the aortic valve approach

A.   Transverse aortotomy
B.   Open aorta exposing the aortic valve

4.5. VALVE ACTION :

4.5.1. Mitral valve :

After performing the left atriotomy, the anterior leaflet of the mitral valve was resected while trying to preserve the posterior leaflet with its cords and ventricular insertions in order to avoid future dilatations of the left ventricle. However, it was not always possible to preserve the posterior leaflet, particularly in the case of extensive calcification of the leaflet, which necessitated complete resection of both leaflets. The prosthesis was fixed in place with intra-annular U-stitches (Figure 6). The anatomical relationships of the mitral valve with the aortic valve, the conduction pathways and the circumflex artery were taken into account when fitting the prosthesis.

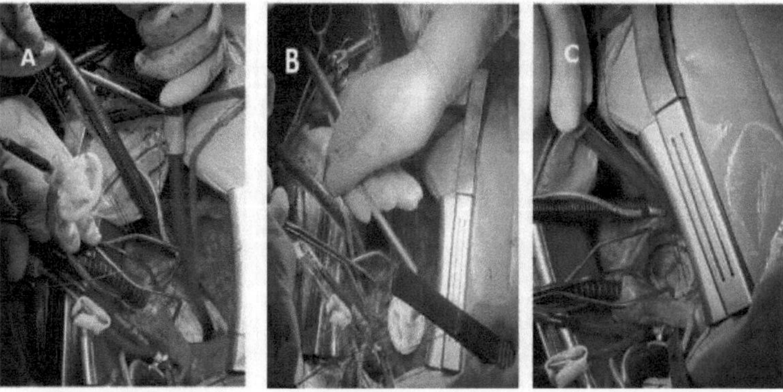

Figure 6: Surgical view of mitral valve replacement with a bioprosthesis

A. Fixation of the bioprosthesis with suspended U-stitches
B. Fixation of the mitral bioprosthesis with intra-annular U-stitches
C. Mitral stent in place

4.5.2. Aortic valve :

After aortotomy, the aortic valve was excised with careful handling of valve calcifications or vegetation depending on the etiology to prevent fragmentation and systemic embolisation of calcareous debris or septic material. The prosthesis was fixed either with "U" stitches, three overjections (Figure 7) or single stitches.

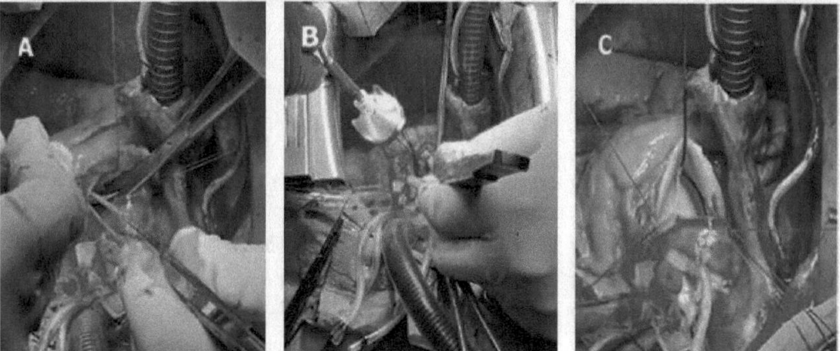

Figure 7: Surgical view of aortic valve replacement with a bioprosthesis

A. Aortic valve resection

B. Fixation of the bioprosthesis with 3 suspended threads C. Placement of the bioprosthesis in the intra-annular position

4.5.3. Tricuspid valve :

After a right atriotomy and verification of the condition of the tricuspid valve, conservative treatment was often possible. In this case, we performed a tricuspid annuloplasty using a rigid ring fixed by U-shaped stitches, while respecting the area of conduction tissue. If the valvular lesions were too extensive, the tricuspid valve was replaced.

The technique we adapted was to use the remnants of the septal valve to suture the bioprosthesis, respecting the area of the anteroseptal commissure and the anterior part of the inner leaflet (Figure 8).

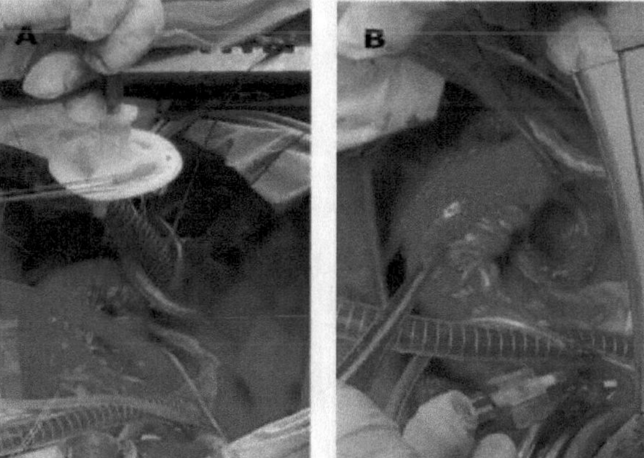

Figure 8: Surgical view of tricuspid valve replacement with a bioprosthesis

A.   Fixation of the bioprosthesis using U points

B.   Intra-annular placement of the bioprosthesis

5. Post-operative evaluation of patients :

5.1. Immediate post-operative care:

All patients were started on a 48-hour _{regeneration} cephalosporin antibiotic prophylaxis and a low-dose acetylsalicylic acid platelet inhibitor. Anticoagulation was resumed at H6 post-op in the absence of bleeding for patients who were already on Acenocoumarol and for patients who had had mitral valve replacement for 3 months. This anticoagulation was ensured by low molecular weight heparin, followed by antivitamin K once the chest tubes had been removed.

The recommendations of the European Society of Cardiology (ESC) recommend curative anticoagulation for three months for bioprostheses in the mitral position (IIa) [4]. For aortic bioprostheses, the surgeon has the choice between effective anticoagulation or platelet anti-aggregation with aspirin for a period of three months (IIb) [4].

We found :

- Length of stay in an intensive care unit
- Intubation time
- The need for repeat surgery for a hemostasis procedure
- Complications arising during hospitalisation (infectious pneumonia, renal failure, post-operative MI, cerebrovascular accident, rhythm or conduction disorders, mediastinitis, etc.).

According to the CDC (Center for Disease Control and Prevention), mediastinitis is defined as an infection of tissues above the subcutaneous level, with or without infection of the retrosternal space, and associated with at least one of the following criteria [8]:

- Sternal instability or fever > 38° C associated with discharge of purulent fluid
- Positive culture of mediastinal tissue or fluid samples
- Obvious mediastinitis on revision surgery (sternal dehiscence/stigmata of infection)
- Length of hospital stay
- Hospital mortality

5.2. Remote post-operative :

We noted the follow-up of patients in the short and medium term. Patients were reviewed daily and before their transfer to cardiology, then at the outpatient clinic between D21 and D30, at 3 months, at 6 months and at 1 year.

All patients were followed up post-operatively and called to complete the interview in order to identify distant post-operative complications, return to work, current activity and sport.

Patients were monitored clinically and by ultrasound. We noted :

- Recurrence of dyspnea and chest pain
- The onset of heart failure
- The following parameters at surveillance ultrasound :
- The trans-prothetical gradient
- The functional surface
- Measuring PAPS
- Measuring EF

6. Statistical analysis :

The data were entered using Microsoft Office 2016 Excel and analysed using SPSS version 25.0 statistical software.

The descriptive study is based on the calculation of means, medians, standard deviations (standard derivations) and range (extreme values = minimum and maximum) for quantitative variables, and on the calculation of absolute frequencies and relative frequencies (percentages) for qualitative variables.

For the analysis of the association between two qualitative variables, the comparison of two frequencies on independent series was carried out by Pearson's Chi2 test in the case of verified conditions of application, and by Fischer's test in the case of non-validity.

For the analysis of the association between a qualitative variable and a quantitative variable, the comparison of two medians was carried out using the non-parametric Mann Whitney test. The comparison of two paired frequencies was carried out using the McNemar paired test if the conditions of application were verified.

Multivariate analysis was performed using a bivariate logistic regression model (selection threshold $p = 0.2$). Risk was calculated as the odds ratio (OR) with a 95% confidence interval (95% CI).

We used the significance level for $p < 5\%$.

7. **Bibliographic research :**

This work was based on a bibliographic search in French and English using the search engines "scholar.google.com", "www.sciencedirect.com" and the PubMed interface using the following keywords in French: chirurgie cardiaque, circulation extracorporelle, bioprothese, valve aortique, valve mitrale, remplacement valvulaire cardiaque.

The key words in English were: cardiac surgery, cardiac pulmonary bypass, bioprosthesis, aortic valve, mitral valve, cardiac valve replacement.

The bibliography was inserted using Zotero software.

8. **Declarations of interest:**

We, the author and supervisor, declare that we have no conflicts of interest in relation to this work. None of us, or any of the patients in the series, has been paid or funded by any pharmaceutical industry.

9. **Ethical considerations:**

Due to the retrospective nature of the study, patients did not sign an informed consent form for the use of personal data contained in the medical records.

Personal data was collected with strict respect for patients' anonymity and the confidentiality of their information.

1. **DESCRIPTIVE STUDY :**

1. **General data :**

Between 1ᵉʳ September 2017 and December 2021, 106 patients had bioprosthesis valve replacement at three cardiovascular surgery centres. 162 patients were not included and 56 records were excluded.

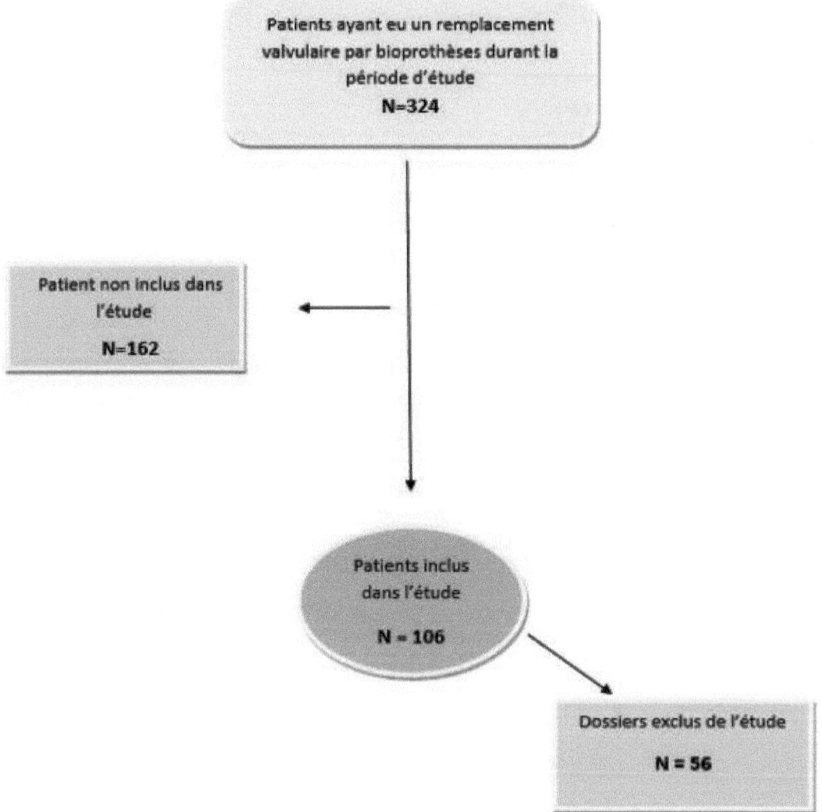

2. **Demographic data :**

2.1. **Age :**

The average age of the patients studied was 68 ± 11.68 years [17-90]. (Figure N°9)

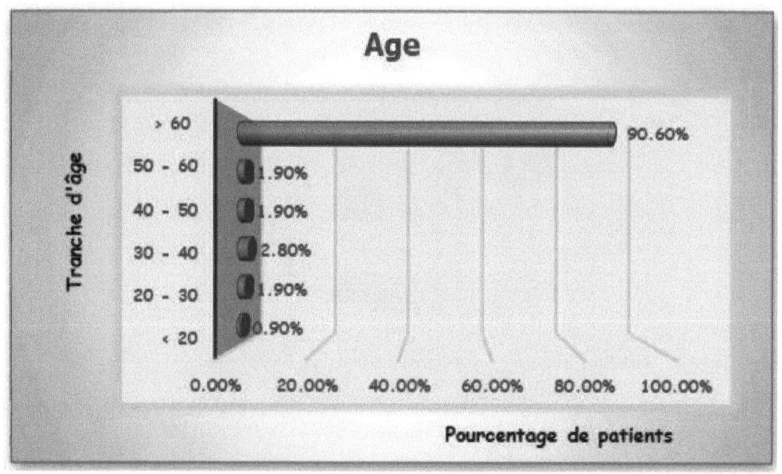

Figure 9: Breakdown of the population by age

Ten of our patients (9%), aged between 17 and 45, opted for a bioprosthesis because of poor compliance with treatment or for professional reasons (Table I).

Table I: Choice of bioprosthesis in the young population

	Age	Choice of bioprosthesis for:	
Patient 1	45	Poor compliance with medication	Prosthesis thrombosis two months after surgery 2ᵉᵐᵉ choice: Bioprosthesis
Patient 2	17	Poor compliance with medication + childbearing age	
Patient 3	35	Poor compliance + Drug addiction	Early endocarditis in prostheses 2ᵉᵐᵉ choice : Bioprosthesis
Patient 4	24	Profession: Sports teacher	
Patient 5	36	Poor compliance with medication	
Patient 6	40	Profession: Policeman	
Patient 7	27	Poor compliance with medication	
Patient 8	30	Poor compliance with medication + desire to become pregnant	
Patient 9	39	Profession: Farmer	
Patient 10	45	Poor compliance with medication	

1.1. Gender:

Of the 106 patients included in the study, 64 were men (61%) and 42 were women (39%), giving a sex ratio of 1.52, with a clear male predominance (Figure 10).

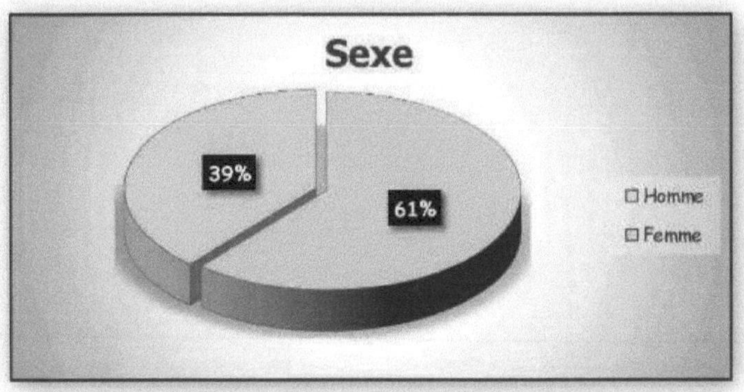

Figure 10: Distribution du sexe selon la fréquence

1.2. Cardiovascular risk factors :

The main cardiovascular risk factors identified in our study are (Figure 11):
- Arterial hypertension: Our series included 59 hypertensive patients (55.7%).
- Smoking: This was found in 44 patients (41.5%).
- Diabetes: There were 25 diabetics (29.2%).
- Dyslipidemia: 31 patients were dyslipidemic (23.6%)
- Obesity: BMI calculations revealed 18 obese patients (27.1%).

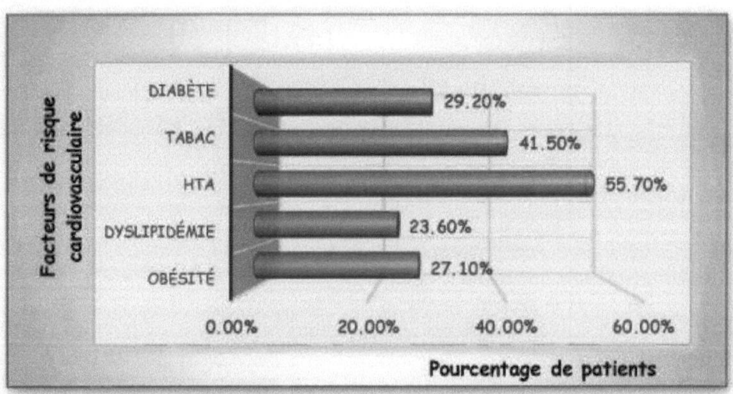

Figure 11: Distribution of patients according to cardiovascular risk factors

1.3. Associated pathologies:

The table below lists the antecedents found in our series:

Table II: Breakdown of patients by medical history

	Fréquence	Pourcentage
Aucun	10	9,4 %
BPCO	44	41,5 %
AVC / AIT	2	1,9 %
Coronaropathie	22	20,7 %
Insuffisance rénale	7	6,6 %
Rhumatisme articulaire aigu	13	12,3 %
Toxicomanie	1	0,9 %

1.4. Previous cardiac surgery :

6.6% of our patients had a history of prior cardiac surgery. Two patients (1.9%) underwent closed-heart mitral commissurotomy. Three patients had a history of mitral valve replacement (2.8%) and three had a history of aortic valve replacement (2.8%).

1.5. Distribution according to etiology :

In our series, degenerative valve disease was predominant. It was present in 55 patients (51.90%), followed by rheumatic pathology in 39 patients (36.8%), then infective endocarditis in eight patients (7.5%).

Other etiologies were less frequent, including aortic bicuspidism in two patients (1.9%), Barlow's disease in three patients (2.8%), ischemic etiology in two patients (1.9%) and systemic lupus erythematosus in a single case (0.9%) (Figure 12).

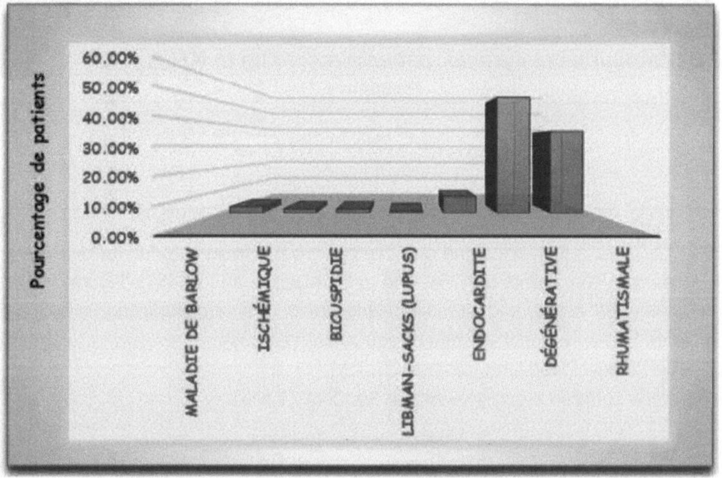

Figure 12: Breakdown of patients by etiology

1.6. Taking medication :

27 patients were on antiplatelet agents (25%) and 39 patients on anticoagulants (36.8%).

1.7. Euroscore II :

The mean predicted patient mortality according to the Euroscore was 2.69% ± 1.17 [0.62% -7%] (Figure 13).

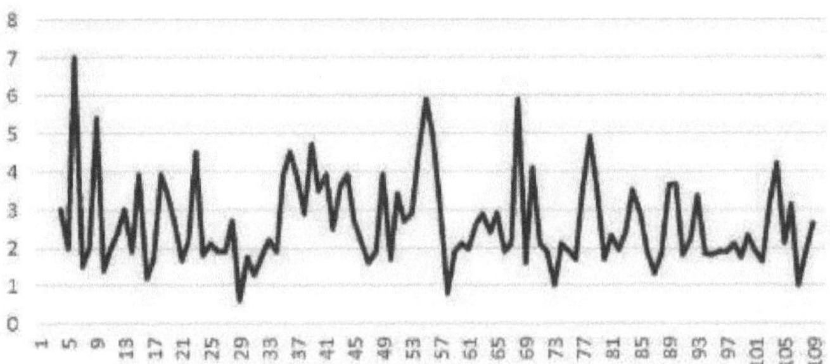

Figure 13: Distribution of patients according to Euroscore II

11. CLINICAL STUDY :

1. Functional signs :

Four patients were asymptomatic (3.8%).

Dyspnea was the functional sign most frequently found in our patients (85 patients, i.e. 80.2%). According to the NYHA (New York Heart Association) classification, patients presented a variable intensity with a predominance of stage III at 53.3% followed by stage II at 39.5%. The following table summarises the distribution of dyspnoeic patients according to NYHA stage.

Table III: Distribution of dyspneic patients according to NYHA stage

	Frequency	Percentage
Stage I	1	1,2 %
Stage II	34	39,5 %
Stage III	45	53,5 %
Stage IV	5	5,8 %

In the other patients, palpitations and chest pain were the main reasons for discovery. Chest pain was present in 40 patients (37.7%) and palpitations in 39 (36.8%) (Figure 14).

The other signs were varied, and were sometimes seen when a complication arose:

- 24 patients had a syncopal episode or equivalent (22.6%).
- Four patients developed limb ischemia (3.8%).
- Two patients suffered a cerebrovascular accident (1.8%).

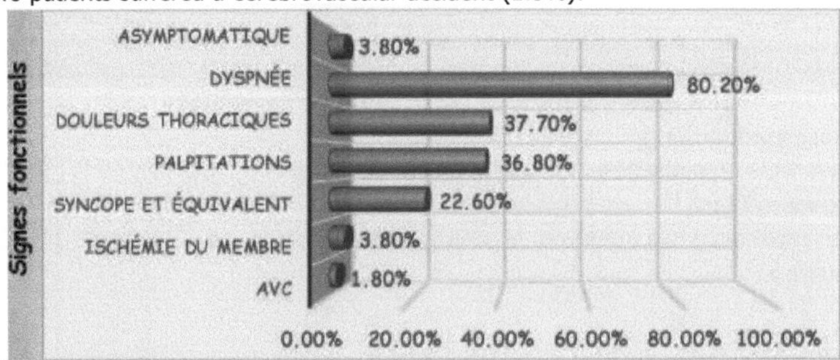

Figure 14: Clinical presentation in patients

2. Physical signs :

Physical examination revealed an auscultatory abnormality at the mitral focus in 26 patients (24.5%) and at the aortic focus in 86 patients (81.1%).
25 patients had heart failure (23.5%).
Two patients presented with coldness and erythrocyanosis of the lower limb in relation to acute ischemiaë (1.8%), two others presented with flaccid hemiplegia secondary to stroke (1.8%) (Figure 15).

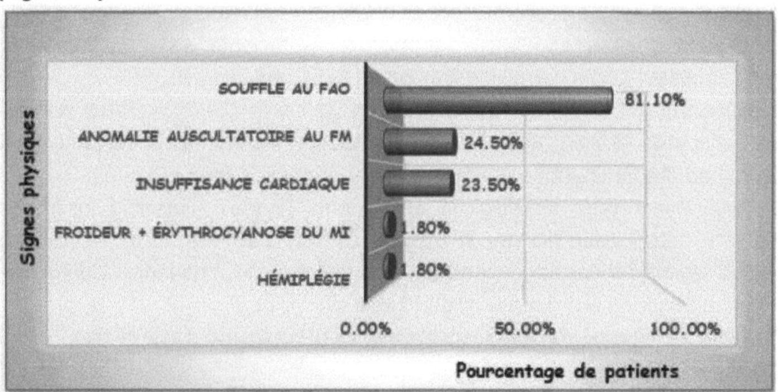

Figure 15: Results of physical examination in patients

3. Additional examinations :

3.1. Chest X-ray:

Chest X-rays were taken in all patients. It was normal in 7 cases and pathological in the 99 others. The various radiological aspects are summarised in Table IV:

Table IV: Distribution of radiological signs in patients

	Frequency	Percentage
Normal	7	6,6 %
Cardiomegaly	49	46,2 %
Mitral silhouette	10	9,4 %
Protrusion of the aortic button	79	74,5 %
Hilar overload	22	20,8 %

3.2. Electrocardiogram (ECG) :

The ECG was normal in 53 patients.
Rhythm disorders were the most frequent electrical signs. Atrial fibrillation was observed in 28 patients.
Eleven patients had conduction disorders.
In addition, 21 patients had repolarisation disorders.
The electrical signs are summarised in Table V.

Table V: Distribution of patients according to electrical signs

	Frequency	Percentage
ECG Normal	53	50 %
Atrial fibrillation	28	26,4 %
Repolarisation disorders	21	19,8 %
Conduction disorders	11	20,8 %

3.3.Echocardiography-doppler :

Transthoracic echocardiography was performed in all patients. The mean LV ejection fraction of the patients was 61% ± 0.08 [35% - 80%]. 97 patients had a preserved left ventricular ejection fraction (91.5%).

The mean pulmonary artery pressure was 36.4% ± 13.35 [18 mmhg - 80 mmhg]. In our study, 24 patients (22.4%) had severe pre-operative PAH.

The left ventricle was dilated in 19 patients (17.9%), while the right ventricle was dilated in seven patients (6.6%). Four patients had biventricular dilatation (3.7%).

Echocardiography showed a predominance of aortic valve disease in 85 patients (80.1%). 27 patients had aortic disease (25.4%). Isolated aortic insufficiency was described in 7 patients (6.6%), while isolated aortic narrowing was noted in 51 patients (48.1%).

Involvement of the mitral valve was observed in 22 cases (20.7%). Mitral narrowing was present in 5 patients (4.7%), while mitral insufficiency was found in 15 patients (14.1%). Two patients had predominantly stenosating mitral disease (1.8%).

Tricuspid involvement was described in 10 patients (9.4%). Tricuspid insufficiency was associated with mitral valve disease in 6 cases (5.6%) and with aortic valve disease in 2 cases (1.8%). Isolated tricuspid involvement was observed in 2 patients (1.8%). The results of the cardiac ultrasound are summarised in Table VI:

Table VI: Distribution of patients according to ultrasound data of the valvulopathies

	Frequency	Percentage
Heart cavities		
LVEF (%)		
> 50	**97**	**91,5 %**
30 < EF < 50	9	8,4 %
HVG	73	68,8 %
Dilatation of the LV	23	21,6 %
Dilatation of the VD	11	10,3 %
Aortic valve	**86**	**81,1 %**
Ao shrinkage	**51**	**48,1 %**
Ao insufficiency	7	6,6 %
Ao disease	**27**	**25,4 %**
Thrombosis of Ao prosthesis	1	0,9 %
Mitral valve	24	26,4 %
Mitral narrowing	5	4,7 %
Mitral insufficiency	**15**	**14,1 %**
Mitral prolapse	9	8,4 %
Mitral disease	2	1,8 %
Mitral prosthesis thrombosis	1	0,9 %
Mitral prosthesis insertion	1	0,9 %
Tricuspid valve	10	9,4 %
IT associated with valvulopathy mitral	**6**	**5,6 %**
IT associated with valvulopathy aortic	2	1,8 %
Isolated tricuspid disease	2	1,8 %
Associated lesions		
Vegetation	9	8,4 %
Thrombus	6	5,6 %
Abces	4	3,7 %

<table>
<tr><td>LVEF= Ventricular ejection fraction</td><td>Left ventricular hypertrophy,</td></tr>
<tr><td>LV= Left Ventricle, LV= Ventricle</td><td>right, Ao= aortic, IT=   Tricuspid insufficiency.</td></tr>
</table>

The majority of patients had single valve disease (84.9%). 16 patients had double valve disease (15%) corresponding to mitro-aortic disease in 8 patients, mitro-tricuspid disease in 6 patients and aorto-tricuspid disease in two patients. No patient had triple valve disease. The distribution of valvular lesions is shown in the table below:

Table VII: Breakdown of valve damage in patients

	Frequency	**Percentage**
Single-valvular disease	90	84,9 %
Mitro-aortic disease	8	7,5 %
Mitro-tricuspid disease	6	5,6 %
Aortotricuspid disease	2	1,8 %

3.4. Coronary angiography :

Preoperative coronary angiography, performed in patients aged over 45 or with cardiovascular risk factors, revealed significant coronary lesions in 21 patients, 11 of whom underwent coronary bypass surgery at the same time (10.4%).

3.5. Echo-doppler data from the supra-aortic trunks:

Doppler ultrasound of the supra-aortic trunks revealed four cases of significant carotid stenosis in patients who were asymptomatic. No patient underwent carotid surgery combined with valve replacement.

4. Operating data :

4.1. Approach :

The thoracic approach was a vertical median sternotomy in 91 patients (85.8%), and a mini-sternotomy in 15 patients (14.1%). The latter was used only for isolated aortic valve replacements.

4.2. Extracorporeal circulation (ECC):

The average duration of bypass surgery was 100.83 ± 33 minutes [34 min - 180 min], while the average duration of aortic clamping was 74.94 ± 41.45 minutes [27 min - 180 min].

In 16 patients (15%) exit from bypass was easy without the use of vasoactive drugs. On the other hand, 53 patients required low doses of catecholamines at the end of the bypass procedure (50%), while 37 patients (35%) underwent the procedure with high doses of catecholamines.

4.3. Surgical procedure:

23 patients underwent emergency surgery (21.7%). The circumstances justifying emergency surgery were numerous and generally related to a complication. These were either cardiac failure, following a syncopal episode or embolic accident, or related to prosthesis dysfunction.

Mitral valve replacement was performed in 26 patients (24.5%). Aortic valve replacement was performed in the majority of the population (86 patients or 81%), while tricuspid valve replacement was performed in 10 patients (9.4%). The different valve replacements are illustrated in Figure 16.

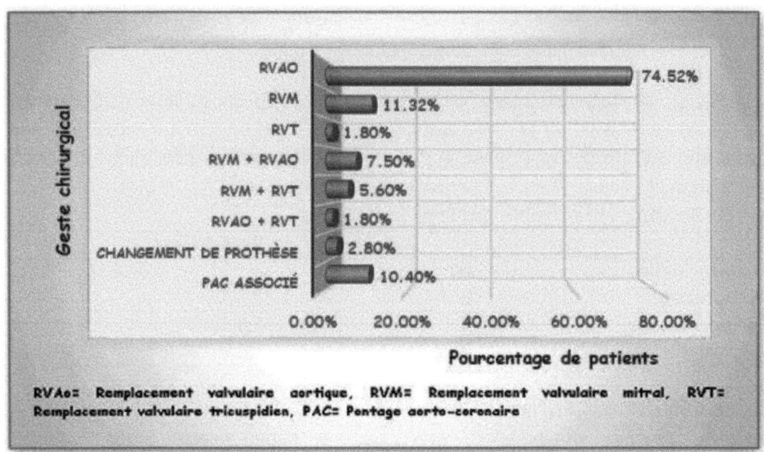

Figure 16: Breakdown of patients by surgical procedure

4.4. Per-operational events :

Out of 106 patients who underwent surgery, 9 (8.4%) developed conduction problems intraoperatively.

Six per-operative deaths were reported as a result of failure to exit the extracorporeal circulation (5.6%).

5. Evolving data :

5.1. Intensive care unit management :

The average length of stay in intensive care was 5 ± 6 days [1-58]. During this period, the average time to extubation was 11 ± 33 hours [0-48]. Total hospital stay was 12 ± 11 days [2-55].

29 patients were weaned off vasoactive drugs in the operating theatre (27%). Weaning of patients was easy with low doses of catecholamines in 40.6% of cases and difficult in 23.6% of cases.

Antibiotic prophylaxis with cephalosporin 1ere generation was systematic for all patients during the first 48 hours. However, curative antibiotic therapy was required in 52 patients (49%) on the basis of clinical, radiological and biological evidence.

56 patients (56%) underwent heparin-based curative anticoagulation to achieve an aPTT of 2.5 - 3.5 times the control. This curative anticoagulation concerned patients with atrial fibrillation and those who had a bioprosthesis in the mitral position.

5.2. Post-operative morbidity and mortality :

5.2.1. Mortality :

In our series, 21 early deaths occurred during the post-operative period, giving a post-operative mortality rate of 19.8%, bringing the total number of deaths to 27 patients and a hospital mortality rate of 25.4%.

The causes of post-operative death were septic shock related to infective pneumonitis in 10 cases (9.4%), infective endocarditis in 3 cases (3%), related to myocardial infarction in one patient, post-operative tamponade in six patients (5%) and cardiogenic shock in one patient (1%). The causes of death are summarised in Table VIII:

Table VIII: Causes of early death

	Frequency	Percentage
IDM	1	1 %

Cardiogenic shock	1	1%	
Post-operative tamponade	6	6 %	
Infectious lung disease	10		10 %
Endocarditis	3	3 %	

5.2.2. Morbidity:

The early post-operative outcome was favourable in 20 patients (20%), while 80 patients developed complications after the operation, giving an overall morbidity of 80%.

5.2.2.1. Complications unrelated to the prosthesis :

■ **Bleeding complications :**

Out of 100 patients who underwent surgery, 24 developed post-operative bleeding, 16 of whom (16%) required further surgery to check their hemostasis. For the other patients, hemostasis disorders were controlled medically and with blood products.

■ **Pulmonary complications :**

The most frequent complications were infectious pneumonitis in 52 patients (49%). The evolution was satisfactory after parental antibiotic therapy and respiratory kinesitherapy in 42 patients (39.6%).

■ **Acute lung injury (OAP):**

The occurrence of post-operative acute lung injury was noted in 17 patients (17%) with a good clinical course with adequate medical treatment and non-invasive ventilation. The causes of PAO were massive transfusion and hypertensive peak.

■ **Post-operative myocardial infarction :**

We noted the occurrence of a documented myocardial infarction during hospitalisation in a single patient who had undergone coronary artery bypass grafting concomitant with valve replacement.

The diagnosis was made on the basis of ECG electrical changes and an increase in troponin levels.

The course of the disease was unfavourable and the patient died despite being put on optimal medical treatment comprising curative dose heparinotherapy and platelet anti-aggregation based on aspirin and Clopidogrel.

■ **Rhythm disorders :**

18 patients (18%) who were in sinus rhythm prior to the operation progressed to atrial fibrillation post-operatively. These patients retained a permanent arrhythmia requiring long-term anticoagulant treatment.

■ **Conduction disorders :**

Seven patients (7%) who had no pre-operative conductive problems developed post-operative atrioventricular block (AVB) 3eme degree. The latter was transient in five patients and permanent in the other two, necessitating the use of a permanent brace.

■ **Post-operative tamponade :**

Eleven (11%) presented with post-operative tamponade, which progressed well after evacuation, with the exception of two patients who died.

■ **Neurological complications :**

In our series, we noted one case of post-operative stroke without sequelae and two cases of post-extubation agitation. These events were documented in patients with no significant pre-operative carotid lesions and no prior cerebral lesions. All three patients had peroperative calcified aortic narrowing, so embolus migration was a likely etiology.

■ **Wall infection :**

Of the 100 patients who underwent surgery, nine (9%) developed post-operative mediastinitis, diagnosed as sternal instability with or without purulent discharge from the surgical wound. Of these nine patients, five were recalled for post-operative bleeding and one was diabetic.

The outcome was satisfactory in 6 patients (6%) after flattening and refixation of the sternum, and fatal in the other three, who went into septic shock.

5.2.2.2. Complications related to the prosthesis :

■ Early endocarditis on prosthesis :

Out of 100 patients operated on, four cases of early endocarditis on prostheses were observed post-operatively (1.9%) in two patients known to be diabetic and in two others admitted with heart failure, one of whom had pre-operative endocarditis on a native valve. One patient had a favourable outcome with appropriate antibiotic therapy. The other three patients required urgent revision surgery for refractory heart failure.

■ Early prosthesis thrombosis :

We noted only one case of early prosthesis thrombosis following interruption of antiaggregant and anticoagulant treatment two months after surgery. The thrombosis was intermittently obstructive (1%) in a mitral prosthesis with a 10 x 14 mm thrombus tilting on either side of the prosthesis. Clinically, the patient had progressively worsening stage II dyspnoea with no evidence of heart failure.

Prior to surgery, the patient opted for a bioprosthesis because of her previous history of poor compliance with anticoagulant therapy for atrial fibrillation. She made the same choice regarding the type of prosthesis before undergoing the same operation again because of her poor compliance with treatment. The post-operative follow-up was straightforward.

Table IX summarises the early complications observed in our series:

Table IX: Distribution of patients according to post-operative complications (n=100):

	Frequency	Percentage
Complications unrelated to the prosthesis :		
Bleeding complications	24	24%
Post-operative bleeding	24	24 %
Reworking for decaillotage	16	16 %
Lung infection	**52**	**52 %**
OAP	17	17 %
IDM	1	1 %
Rhythm disorder	18	18 %
Conduction disorder	7	7 %
BAV 3rd transitional	5	5%
BAV 3rd permanent	2	2%
Tamponade	11	11 %
Neurological complications	3	3 %
Mediastinitis	9	9 %
Complications related to the prosthesis :		
Early endocarditis	4	4 %
Obstructive thrombosis	1	1 %

OAP= acute pulmonary oedema, MI= myocardial infarction

6. Follow-up:

Of the 100 patients who survived the hospital period, only 66 (66%) could be contacted. Difficulties encountered during patient follow-up were mostly due to missing or invalid contact details. The patients contacted were checked clinically and ultrasonographically.

The average follow-up time from the last consultation was 54.5 months, with extremes of six to 70 months.

6.1. Clinical course :

We found that dyspnoea disappeared in 56 patients (84.8%) and improved in eight others (12.1%), moving from NHYA stage III to stage II.

Patients who had syncope pre-operatively did not have a syncopal episode after the operation. Two patients (3%) who had cardiac decompensation pre-operatively retained signs of heart failure.

6.2. Ultrasound evolution :

6.2.1. patients were rechecked by echocardiography. The time between surgery and echocardiography ranged from six to 66 months. The parameters studied were :

6.2.2. The prothetic profile :

Echocardiography revealed a good hemodynamic profile for the implanted bioprostheses in 90.9% of cases (60 patients reviewed). Three patients had a stenosing bioprosthesis at a distance (4%) and two others had a leaky prosthesis (3%).

The three patients with a stenosante bioprosthesis all had aortic bioprostheses, N°19 in two cases and N°21 in one case. A mismatch would be likely given the relatively small effective surface area for these bioprostheses. These patients were asymptomatic and were monitored closely with optimisation of anticoagulation in cases of stenosis of the prosthesis. None of these patients were re-staged within the time frame of the study. For patients with a leaking bioprosthesis, the leak was central with a grade 1 to 2 insufficiency. These patients were asymptomatic and no worsening was noted during iterative ultrasound controls.

Table X shows the type of replacement, size and brand of prosthesis associated with these five cases of prosthetic complications.

Table X: Prothetic profile after ultrasound examination

Patient N°	Type of replacement	Size of prosthesis (mm)	Brand of prosthesis	Profile prothetics
76	Aortic	21	Crown (Sorin)	Stenosant
78	Aortic	19	Crown (Sorin)	Stenosant
83	Aortic	19	Trifecta	Stenosant
98	Aortic	21	Crown (Sorin)	Running away
105	Mitral	31	Pericarbon More	Running away

6.2.3. Systolic pulmonary arterial pressure (SPAP) :

The mean control PAPS was 32.59 ± 11.75 mmhg [20 - 80].

Improvement in pulmonary arterial hypertension (PAH) was observed in 24 patients (36.6%).

40 patients (60.6%) maintained the same preoperative pulmonary pressures and two worsened their PAH.

6.2.4. Ejection fraction (EF) :

The mean control EF was 52 ± 0.08% [35 and 70%].

6.2.5. Left ventricular hypertrophy (LVH) :

34 patients (51.5%) retained LVH on ultrasound examination, while 11 patients (16.6%) who had pre-operative LVH did not.

6.2.6. Intra-auricular thrombus :

Of the 66 patients who had a follow-up echocardiogram, intra-atrial thrombus was detected in six (9%), three of whom had stenosing prostheses.

6.3.Late mortality:

In the series studied, only one late death was reported by the family, with no specific cause.

111. STATISTICAL STUDY :

1. Factors predictive of morbidity :

In this study, we compared the pre-, intra- and post-operative data for 100 patients who had not been discharged intraoperatively, with regard to the occurrence of complications and mortality.

1.1.Epidemiological factors :

Post-operative complications were significantly associated with body mass index (p=0.013). They were observed in all patients with a history of coronary artery disease (p=0.021), were more marked in male patients, and in patients with rheumatic pathology (OR > 1), with no significant association.

Table XI shows the epidemiological factors associated with post-operative morbidity:

Table XI: Epidemiological factors associated with post-operative morbidity

C	COMPLICATIONS (n = 84)	NO COMPLICATIONS (n = 16)	p	OR [95% CI]
Age (years)	71,5 [67-73]	70 [68-73,5]	0,966	-
BMI (Kg/m)^2	27,11 [26-28]	28,7 [27,3-30,4]	**0,013**	-
Weight insufficiency	2 (100%)	0 (0%)	0,404	-
Normal	3 (100%)	0 (0%)	0,302	-
Overweight	27 (75%)	9 (25%)	1	1 [0,221-4,521]
Obesite	4 (57,1%)	3 (42,9%)	0,238	0,375 [0,071-1,991]
Type				
Male	56 (88,9%)	7 (11,1%)	0,082	2,571 [0,867-7,625]
Female	28 (75,7%)	9 (24,3%)		0,389 [0,131-1,153]
Treatment in progress	26 (83,9%)	5 (16,1%)	0,981	0,986 [0,311-3,127]
Aspegic	21 (87,5%)	3 (12,5%)	0,592	1,444 [0,375-5,566]
Insulin	7 (77,8%)	2 (22,2%)	0,594	0,636 [0,12-3,385]
Medical history and FRCVs	78 (83%)	16 (17%)	0,27	-
Rheumatic diseases	11 (84,6%)	2 (15,4%)	0,948	1,055 [0,211-5,285]
Diabetes	18 (75%)	6 (25%)	0,168	0,455 [0,146-1,419]
Tobacco	36 (83,7%)	7 (16,3%)	0,947	0,964 [0,328-2,834]
HTA	44 (80%)	11 (20%)	0,228	0,5 [0,16-1,564]
Dyslipidemia	22 (75,9%)	7 (24,1%)	0,156	0,456 [0,152-1,372]
Coronary artery disease	21 (100%)	0 (0%)	**0,021**	-
Endocarditis	7 (100%)	0 (0%)	0,231	-
COPD	5 (100%)	0 (0%)	0,317	-
AVC	2 (100%)	0 (0%)	0,533	-
IRC	5 (71,4%)	2 (28,6%)	0,347	0,443 [0,078-2,513]
Hemodialysis	4 (80%)	1 (20%)	0,802	0,75 [0,078-7,185]
Drug addiction	1 (100%)	0 (0%)	0,661	-
Previous cardiac surgery	5 (83,3%)	1 (16,7%)	0,963	0,949 [0,103-8,714]
RVAo	1 (50%)	1 (50%)	0,121	-
RVM	3 (100%)	0 (0%)	0,273	-
CMCF	1 (100%)	0 (0%)	0,624	-

FRCV= Risk factors cardiovascular, AVR= Aortic Valve Replacement, MVR= Mitral valve replacement, CMCF=Commissurotomy of the mitral valve with closed heart

1.2.Pre-operational factors :

1.2.1. Clinical data :

No clinical factors were associated with post-operative morbidity. Post-operative complications were more frequently observed in the context of urgent management and in the presence of syncope and equivalent (OR > 1), with no significant difference.

Table XII illustrates the clinical factors associated with post-operative morbidity:

Table XII: Clinical factors associated with post-operative morbidity

	COMPLICATIONS (n = 84)	NO COMPLICATIONS (n = 16)	p	OR [95% CI]
Euroscore	2,25 [1,9-3,5]	2,05 [1,8-2,8]	0,421	-
Emergency context	17 (85%)	3 (15%)	0,892	1,1 [0,281-4,299]
Response time (months)	7 [3-12]	11 [2,5-20]	0,428	-
Etiology				
Rheumatic	30 (83,3%)	6 (16,7%)	0,892	0,926 [0,306-2,799]
Degenerative	43 (81,1%)	10 (18,9%)	0,406	0,629 [0,21-1,888]
Endocarditis	7 (100%)	0 (0%)	0,231	-
LibmanSacks Lupus	1 (100%)	0 (0%)	0,661	-
Bicuspidia	2 (100%)	0 (0%)	0,533	-
Hypertensive heart disease	2 (66,7%)	1 (33,3%)	0,406	0,366 [0,031-4,294]
Ischemic	2 (100%)	0 (0%)	0,533	-
Barlow's disease	3 (100%)	0 (0%)	0,443	-
Clinical signs				
Dyspnea	66 (82,5%)	14 (17,5%)	0,413	0,524 [0,109-2,519]
NYHA II	27 (84,4%)	5 (15,6%)	0,719	1,246 [0,376-4,13]
NYHA III	36 (83,7%)	7 (16,3%)	0,757	1,2 [0,378-3,806]
NYHA IV	3 (60%)	2 (40%)	0,209	0,286 [0,043-1,896]
Heart failure	19 (82,6%)	4 (17,4%)	0,836	0,877 [0,253-3,035]
Syncope and equivalent	20 (90,9%)	2 (9,1%)	0,317	2,188 [0,458-10,45]
Chest pain	35 (89,7%)	4 (10,3%)	0,21	2,143 [0,638-7,2]
Embolic event	4 (100%)	0 (0%)	0,373	-
Vascular purpura	1 (100%)	0 (0%)	0,661	-

1.2.2. Paraclinical data :

Post-operative complications predominated in all patients with atrial fibrillation on ECG (p=0.005) and in all patients with left ventricular dilatation on echocardiography (p=0.021).

They were more frequent in patients with mitral silhouette on chest X-ray, conduction and repolarisation disorders on ECG, significant coronary lesions on coronary angiography, left ventricular hypertrophy and mitral insufficiency on ultrasound (OR > 1).

All the associated valve lesions found on ultrasound (vegetations, abscesses, thrombus) were accompanied by post-operative complications. The paraclinical data are summarised in Table XIII :

Table XIII: Paraclinical factors associated with post-operative morbidity

	COMPLICATIONS (n = 84)	NO COMPLICATIONS (n = 16)	p	OR [95% CI]
Chest X-ray				
Cardiomegaly	39 (84,8%)	7 (15,2%)	0,844	1,114 [0,38-3,271]
Hilar overload	16 (80%)	4 (20%)	0,585	0,706 [0,201-2,478]
Mitral silhouette	7 (87,5%)	1 (12,5%)	0,778	1,364 [0,156-11,908]
ECG				
FA	27 (100%)	0 (0%)	**0,005**	-
Conduction disorder	10 (90,9%)	1 (9,1%)	0,508	2,027 [0,241-17,044]

	COMPLICATIONS	NO COMPLICATIONS	p	OR [95% CI]
Repolarisation disorder	16 (88,9%)	2 (11,1%)	0,532	1,647 [0,34-7,985]
Coronary angiography				
Significant lesion	18 (94,7%)	1 (5,3%)	0,156	4,091 [0,506-33,083]
Associated bypass	9 (100%)	0 (0%)	0,17	-
EDTSA				
Significant lesion	4 (100%)	0 (0%)	0,373	-
Ultrasound				
General parameters	4 (100%)	0 (0%)	0,373	-
EF (%)	60 [55-65]	60 [60-65]	0,328	-
PAPS (mmHg)	32 [27-42]	32 [30-36]	0,694	-
HVG	58 (84,1%)	11 (15,9%)	0,981	1,014 [0,32-3,215]
Dilatation of the LV	21 (100%)	0 (0%)	**0,021**	-
Dilatation of the VD	9 (100%)	0 (0%)	0,17	-
Aortic valve				
Initial Ao diameter (mm)	31,5 [29-34]	30 [26,5-32,5]	0,366	-
SAo (cm)^2	0,8 [0,6-0,9]	0,7 [0,6-0,9]	0,839	-
Ao shrinkage	62 (82,7%)	13 (17,3%)	0,529	0,65 [0,169-2,499]
Mean LV-Ao Gdt (mmHg)	49,5 [40-61]	48 [45-59]	0,707	-
Ao insufficiency	28 (82,4%)	6 (17,6%)	0,747	0,833 [0,275-2,526]
Mitral valve				
Prosthesis insertion	1 (100%)	0 (0%)	0,661	-
Mitral narrowing	4 (80%)	1 (20%)	0,802	0,75 [0,078-7,185]
Mitral insufficiency	15 (88,2%)	2 (11,8%)	0,601	1,522 [0,312-7,413]
Mitral prolapse	7 (77,8%)	2 (22,2%)	0,594	0,636 [0,12-3,385]
Associated valve lesions				
Vegetations	8 (100%)	0 (0%)	0,198	-
Abces	4 (100%)	0 (0%)	0,373	-
Thrombus	6 (100%)	0 (0%)	0,27	-

AF= Atrial Fibrillation, EF= Ejection Fraction, PAPS= Systolic Pulmonary Artery Pressure, LVH= Left Ventricular Hypertrophy, LV= Left Ventricle, RV= Right Ventricle, Ao= Aorta, SAo= Aortic Surface, LV-Ao mean Gdt= LV-Ao mean Gradient.

1.3.Intraoperative factors :

We studied the different parameters collected according to the occurrence of postoperative complications (Table XIV). These were significantly more frequent when high doses of catecholamine were required (96.8% vs 77.4%; p=0.026; OR=8.78).

We found that the administration of catecholamines intraoperatively, the use of a mini-sternotomy as an approach, and mitral and tricuspid valve replacements were more incriminated in the occurrence of post-operative complications (OR > 1).

A longer median duration of bypass surgery and aortic clamping was more associated with the occurrence of post-operative complications.

Table XIV: Factors in intraoperative management associated with post-operative morbidity

	COMPLICATIONS (n = 84)	NO COMPLICATIONS (n = 16)	p	OR [95% CI]
Clamping time (min)	69 [51-94,5]	60 [47-74]	0,158	-
CEC time (min)	94,5 [74,5-125,5]	78,5 [72,5-92]	0,055	-
Catecholamines (intra-operative)	71 (84,5%)	13 (15,5%)	0,743	1,26 [0,315-5,048]

Low dose	41 (77,4%)	12 (22,6%)	**0,026**	0,114 [0,014-0,924]
High dose	30 (96,8%)	1 (3,2%)	**0,026**	8,78 [1,082-71,248]
Approach				
Median vertical sternotomy	71 (83,5%)	14 (16,5%)	0,76	0,78 [0,158-3,846]
Mini-sternotomy	13 (86,7%)	2 (13,3%)	0,76	1,282 [0,26-6,318]
Type of VR				
RVM				2,484
	22 (91,7%)	2 (8,3%)	0,24	[0,522-11,813]
RVAo	68 (82,9%)	14 (17,1%)	0,532	0,607 [0,125-2,943]
RVT	6 (85,7%)	1 (14,3%)	0,889	1,169 [0,131-10,424]

CEC= Extracorporeal circulation, RV= Valve replacement, RVM= Mitral valve replacement, RVAo= Aortic valve replacement, RVT= Tricuspid valve replacement.

2. Predictors of mortality :

We will study the mortality rate for 93 patients (87.7%), broken down as follows:

2.1. 6 patients decomposed per-operatively and in the immediate post-operative period.

2.2. 21 patients died during the first 30 days after the operation.

2.3. 66 patients followed up one year after surgery

Only one case of long-term death was reported by the family and not explained, giving a crude mortality rate of 34.6% (n=28). Figure 17 summarises the evolutionary aspect of the population studied.

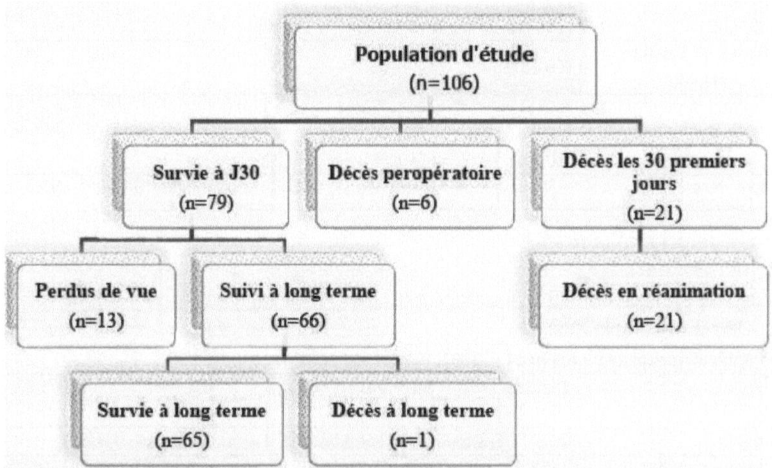

Figure 17: Evolutionary aspect of the population studied

2.4. Epidemiological factors :

Mortality was significantly higher in overweight patients (p= 0.07; OR = 16.7) and in female patients (50% vs 26.4%; p= 0.034; OR = 2.78) (Table XV).

Table XV: Epidemiological factors associated with mortality				
	Deaths (n = 28)	Survival (n = 53)	P	OR	95% CI
Age (years)	72 [69,5-74]	72 [69,5-74]	0,446	-	-
BMI (Kg/m)^2	27,7 [26,1-29,2]	27,7 [26,1-29,2]	0,589	-	-
Weight insufficiency	0 (0%)	0 (0%)	0,171	-	-
Normal	0 (0%)	0 (0%)	0,088	-	-

	Deaths	Survival	p	OR	95% CI
Overweight	13 (65%)	13 (65%)	**0,007**	16,714	1,742-160,35
Obesite	1 (20%)	1 (20%)	0,19	-	-
Type					
Male	14 (26,4%)	14 (26,4%)	**0,034**	0,359	0,137-0,938
Female	14 (50%)	14 (50%)	**0,034**	2,786	1,067-7,276
Treatment in progress	13 (44,8%)	13 (44,8%)	0,147	-	-
Aspegic	9 (40,9%)	9 (40,9%)	0,464	-	-
Insulin	4 (44,4%)	4 (44,4%)	0,509	-	-
Medical history and FRCVs	27 (35,5%)	27 (35,5%)	0,479	-	-
Rheumatic diseases	3 (33,3%)	3 (33,3%)	0,934	-	-
Diabetes	6 (30%)	6 (30%)	0,621	-	-
Tobacco	13 (35,1%)	13 (35,1%)	0,922	-	-
HTA	17 (37%)	17 (37%)	0,604	-	-
Dyslipidemia	7 (29,2%)	7 (29,2%)	0,507	-	-
Coronary artery disease	10 (50%)	10 (50%)	0,094	-	-
Endocarditis	4 (57,1%)	4 (57,1%)	0,189	-	-
COPD	2 (50%)	2 (50%)	0,506	-	-
AVC	0 (0%)	0 (0%)	0,298	-	-
IRC	1 (16,7%)	1 (16,7%)	0,338	-	-
Hemodialysis	0 (0%)	0 (0%)	0,093	-	-
Drug addiction	1 (100%)	1 (100%)	0,166	-	-
History of cardiac surgery	4 (66,7%)	4 (66,7%)	0,086	-	-
RVAo	1 (50%)	1 (50%)	0,54	-	-
RVM	2 (66,7%)	2 (66,7%)	1	-	-
CMCF	2 (100%)	2 (100%)	0,221	-	-

BMI=Body Mass Index, CVRF=Cardiovascular Risk Factors, CKD=Chronic Kidney Disease, AVR=Aortic Valve Replacement, MVR=Mitral Valve Replacement, FMC=Firm Heart Mitral Commissurotomy.

2.5.Pre-operational factors :

2.5.1. Clinical data :

Mortality was significantly higher for procedures performed in an emergency setting (p= 0.011; OR= 3.66) (Table XVI).

Table XVI: Clinical factors associated with mortality

	Deaths (n = 28)	Survival (n = 53)	p	OR	95% CI
Euroscore	2,03 [1,6-2,8]	2,3 [1,9-3,5]	0,151	-	-
Emergency context	12 (57,1%)	9 (42,9%)	**0,011**	3,667	1,301-10,338
Response time (months)	3,5 [2-7,5]	8 [5-12]	**0,016**	-	-
Etiology					
Rheumatic	6 (23,1%)	20 (76,9%)	0,135	-	-
Degenerative	17 (37%)	29 (63%)	0,604	-	-
Endocarditis	4 (57,1%)	3 (42,9%)	0,189	-	-
Libman Sacks Lupus	0 (0%)	1 (100%)	0,465	-	-
Bicuspidia	1 (100%)	0 (0%)	0,166	-	-
Hypertensive heart disease	1 (100%)	0 (0%)	0,166	-	-
Ischemic	2 (100%)	0 (0%)	0,117	-	-
Barlow's disease	1 (50%)	1 (50%)	0,642	-	-
Clinical signs					
Dyspnea	25 (37,9%)	41 (62,1%)	0,189	-	-
NYHA II	13 (48,1%)	14 (51,9%)	0,152	-	-

	Deaths (n = 28)	Survival (n = 53)	P	OR	95% CI
NYHA III	11 (31,4%)	24 (68,6%)	0,251	-	-
NYHA IV	1 (25%)	3 (75%)	1	-	-
Heart failure	8 (36,4%)	14 (63,6%)	0,836	-	-
Syncope and equivalent	9 (40,9%)	13 (59,1%)	0,464	-	-
Chest pain	11 (36,7%)	19 (63,3%)	0,761	-	-
Embolic event	2 (50%)	2 (50%)	0,506	-	-
Vascular purpura	1 (100%)	0 (0%)	0,166	-	-

2.5.2. Paraclinical data :

Mortality was significantly lower in patients with aortic insufficiency (p= 0.041; OR= 0.298) (Table XVII).

Table XVII: Paraclinical factors associated with mortality

	Deaths (n = 28)	Survival (n = 53)	P	OR	95% CI
Chest X-ray					
Cardiomegaly	12 (32,4%)	25 (67,6%)	0,711	-	-
Hilar overload	9 (52,9%)	8 (47,1%)	0,073	-	-
Double contour	4 (57,1%)	3 (42,9%)	0,189	-	-
ECG					
FA	7 (31,8%)	15 (68,2%)	0,751	-	-
Conduction disorder	6 (54,5%)	5 (45,5%)	0,134	-	-
Repolarisation disorder	8 (53,3%)	7 (46,7%)	0,09	-	-
Coronary angiography					
Significant lesion	10 (52,6%)	9 (47,4%)	0,058	-	-
Associated bypass	5 (50%)	5 (50%)	0,273	-	-
EDTSA					
Significant lesion	0 (0%)	4 (100%)	0,136	-	-
Ultrasound					
General parameters					
EF (%)	61,5 [60-65]	60 [55-65]	0,245	-	-
PAPS (mmHg)	31,5 [28-50]	30 [25-35,5]	0,072	-	-
HVG	21 (36,8%)	36 (63,2%)	0,507	-	-
Dilatation of the LV	7 (41,2%)	10 (58,8%)	0,519	-	-
Dilatation of the VD	5 (55,6%)	4 (44,4%)	0,16	-	-
Aortic valve					
Initial Ao diameter (mm)	32 [25-33]	30 [29-32]	0,838	-	-
SAo (cm)^2	0,84 [0,5-0,9]	0,7 [0,6-0,9]	0,979	-	-
Ao shrinkage	18 (29,5%)	43 (70,5%)	0,094	-	-
Mean LV-Ao Gdt (mmHg)	52,5 [40-68]	47 [42-55]	0,202	-	-
Ao insufficiency	4 (17,4%)	19 (82,6%)	**0,041**	0,298	0,09-0,988
Mitral valve					
Prosthesis insertion	1 (100%)	0 (0%)	0,166	-	-
Mitral narrowing	3 (60%)	2 (40%)	0,217	-	-
Mitral insufficiency	6 (46,2%)	7 (53,8%)	0,338	-	-
Mitral prolapse	4 (57,1%)	3 (42,9%)	0,189	-	-
Associated valve lesions					
Vegetations	5 (62,5%)	3 (37,5%)	0,08	-	-
Abces2 (66.7%)	1 (33.3%)	0.	234--		
Thrombus	3 (50%)	3 (50%)	0, 409-	:	

AF= Atrial Fibrillation, EF= Ejection Fraction, PAPS= Systolic Pulmonary Artery Pressure, LVH= Left Ventricular Hypertrophy, LV= Left Ventricle, RV= Right Ventricle, Ao= Aorta, SAo= Aortic Surface, LV-

Ao mean Gdt= LV-Ao mean Gradient.

2.6.Intraoperative factors :

Mortality was significantly associated with the introduction of vasoactive drugs intraoperatively (p= 0.007). Patients who had difficulty being withdrawn from extracorporeal circulation on high doses of catecholamines had the highest mortality (p<0.001; OR=7.97). We found that patients who had aortic valve replacement had lower mortality than those who had mitral valve replacement, with a statistically significant difference (p = 0.018; OR= 0.274). Table XVIII summarises the per-operative factors associated with mortality:

Table XVIII: Per-operative factors associated with mortality

	Deaths (n = 28)	Survival (n = 53)	p	OR	95% CI
Clamping time (min)	67,5 [46-92,5]	62 [49-79]	0,891	-	-
CEC time (min)	90 [65-152,5]	86 [72-104]	0,644	-	-
Catecholamines (intra-operative)	25 (37,9%)	41 (62,1%)	**0,007**	-	-
Low dose	7 (18,4%)	31 (81,6%)	**<0,001**	0,125	0,041-0,387
High dose	18 (64,3%)	10 (35,7%)	**<0,001**	7,971	2,583-24,604
Approach					
Median vertical sternotomy	28 (41,8%)	39 (58,2%)	**0,002**		
Mini-sternotomy	0 (0%)	14 (100%)	**0,002**		
Type of VR					
RVM	10 (52,6%)	9 (47,4%)	0, 058--		
RVAo	18 (28,1%)	46 (71,9%)	**0,018**	0,2740	,09-0,83
RVT	3 (50%)	3 (50%)	0,409		

CEC= Extracorporeal circulation, RV= Valve replacement, RVM= Mitral valve replacement, RVAo= Aortic valve replacement, RVT= Tricuspid valve replacement.

2.7.Factors related to post-operative management

The length of stay in intensive care and the length of hospitalisation were longer in decedent patients, with no significant association (Table XIX).

Table XIX: Mortality in relation to length of stay in intensive care and length of hospitalisation

	Deaths (n=28)	Survival (n=53)	p
Length of stay in intensive care (days)	8 [5-11]	3 [2-5]	0.73
Length of stay	15 [12-34]	12 [8-18]	0.269

Mortality was significantly associated with the occurrence of tamponade as an immediate postoperative complication (66.7%; p=0.016; OR=6.25). Infectious pneumonitis was associated with a 34.4% mortality with no significant association (Table XX).

Table XX: Post-operative factors associated with mortality

	Deaths (n=28)	Survival (n=53)	P	OR	95% CI
Cardiac Complications					
ACFA	4 (15.4%)	22 (84,6%)	0.053		
BAV	2 (28.6%)	5 (71.4%)		1	
Hypertensive peak	3 (13.6%)	19 (86.4%)	0.054		
Endocarditis	3 (75%)	1 (25%)	0.203		
Valve thrombosis	0 (0%)	1 (100%)		1	
IDM	*1 (100%)*	0 (0%)	0.293		
Tamponade	6 (66.7%)	3 (33.3%)	**0.016**		**6.21.4-27.895**

Pulmonary				
Lung infection	10 (24.4%)	34 (65.6%)	0.302	
OAP	4 (26.7%)	11 (73.3%)		1
Neurological (stroke)	1 (50%)	1 (50%)	0.503	
Mediastinitis	3 (33.3%)	6 (66.7%)	0.716	

3. MULTIVARIATE ANALYTICAL STUDY :

The independent factors of post-operative morbidity and mortality were identified by adjusting the results for patients aged over 70, medical history and associated coronary surgery, as well as the emergency context of the operation.
surgical procedure.

3.1. Independent factors associated with morbidity :

The use of catecholamines was the only independent factor for post-operative morbidity in our study ($p = 0.043$; 11.76) (Table XXI).

Table XXI: Independent factors associated with morbidity

	n (%)	P	OR	95% CI
FA	27 (100%)	-	-	-
Significant coronary lesions	18 (94,7%)	0,161	4,681	0,54-40,57
Associated bypasses	9 (100%)	-	-	-
LV dilation	21 (100%)	-	-	-
VD dilation	9 (100%)	-	-	-
Vegetations	8 (100%)	-	-	-
Low dose	41 (77,4%)	**0,043**	0,085	0,008-0,926
High dose	30 (96,8%)	**0,043**	11,764	1,08-128,12

AF= Atrial Fibrillation, LV= Left Ventricle, RV= Right Ventricle

3.2. Independent factors associated with mortality :

In a multivariate study, the predictive factors for mortality were administration of high-dose catecholamines, with a p of 0.001 and an OR of 10.76, and pulmonary complications, with a p of 0.042 and an OR of 85.8.

Table XXII shows the independent factors associated with mortality:

Table XXII: Independent factors associated with mortality

	n (%)	p	OR	95% CI
Causes				
Rheumatic	6 (23,1%)	0,094	0,316	0,082-1,216
Endocarditis	4 (57,1%)	0,122	7,513	0,584-96,592
Bicuspidia	1 (100%)	-		--
Hypertensive heart disease	1 (100%)	-		--
Ischemic	2 (100%)	-		--
Clinical signs				
Dyspnea	25 (37,9%)	0,526	1,67	0,342-8,16
Vascular purpura	1 (100%)	-	-	-
Chest X-ray				
Hilar overload	9 (52,9%)	0,294	2,001	0,548-7,306
Double contour	4 (57,1%)	0,09	6,437	0,746-55,575
ECG				
Conduction disorder	6 (54,5%)	0,125	3,209	0,722-14,258
Repolarisation disorder	8 (53,3%)	0,593	1,464	0,363-5,907

Coronary angiography				
Significant lesion	10 (52,6%)	0,187	2,319	0,664-8,092
Echocardiography				
VD dilation	5 (55,6%)	0,072	6,233	0,847-45,86
Aortic narrowing	18 (29,5%)	0,388	0,579	0,168-1,998
Aortic insufficiency	4 (17,4%)	0,357	0,542	0,147-1,995
Mitral prosthesis insertion	1 (100%)	-	-	■
Mitral prolapse	4 (57,1%)	0,241	2,988	0,479-18,652
Vegetations	5 (62,5%)	0,111	7,734	0,624-95,837
Operative management				
Catecholamines	25 (37,9%)	-		--
Low dose	7 (18,4%)	**0,001**	0,093	0,021-0,401
High dose	18 (64,3%)	**0,001**	10,765	2,491-46,519
Approach				
Median vertical sternotomy	28 (41,8%)	-		--
Mini-sternotomy	0 (0%)	-		--
Type of VR				
RVM	10 (52,6%)	0,42	1,706	0,465-6,258
RVAo	18 (28,1%)	0,137	0,37	0,1-1,371
Post-operative complications				
ACFA	4 (15,4%)	0.209		
Hypertensive peak	3 (13,6%)	0.112		
Tamponade		6 (66,7%)	0.703	
Pulmonary complications		10 (22,2%)	**0.042**	85.8
Bleeding complications		9 (42,9%)	0.427	
Endocarditis		3 (75%)	0.231	

RV= Right ventricle, RVM= Mitral valve replacement, RVAo= Aortic valve replacement.

5 DISCUSSION

I. SUMMARY OF THE MAIN RESULTS :

We conducted a multicentre retrospective study from September 2017 to December 2021 involving 106 patients who had undergone valve replacement with a bioprosthesis in any position, at the cardiovascular surgery departments of the Abderrahman Mami University Hospital in Ariana, the Habib Bourguiba Hospital in Sfax, and the main military training hospital in Tunis.

The average age of the patients included in the study was 68, with an estimated 9% aged between 17 and 45.

Degenerative valvulopathy predominated in 55 patients (51.90%), followed by rheumatic pathology in 39 patients (36.8%), then infective endocarditis in 8 patients (7.5%).

Aortic valve disease was predominant in 85 patients (80.1%). Mitral valve disease was observed in 22 cases (20.7%). Tricuspid involvement was described in 10 patients (9.4%).

Significant coronary lesions were found in 21 patients, 11 of whom had coronary bypass surgery concomitant with valve surgery (10.4%).

23 patients underwent emergency surgery (21.7%). The circumstances justifying emergency surgery were multiple and generally related to a complication.

The mean duration of bypass surgery was 100.83 ± 33 minutes [34 min - 180 min] and the mean duration of aortic clamping was 74.94 ± 41.45 minutes [27 min - 180 min].

Out of 106 patients operated on, six per-operative deaths were reported (5.6%).

The mean length of stay in intensive care was 5 ± 6 days [1-58]. Total hospital stay was 12 ± 11 days [2-55].

Out of 100 patients operated on, 24 developed post-operative bleeding, 16 of whom (16%) required repeat surgery to check hemostasis.

18 patients (18%) who were in sinus rhythm before the operation went into atrial fibrillation post-operatively, and seven patients (7%) who had no conductive problems pre-operatively developed atrioventricular block (AVB) 3eme post-operatively. Two patients were fitted with devices for definitive 3eme degree AVB, while the conductive disorders regressed in the other five.

We noted 54% infectious pneumonitis, 17% acute lung injury, 11% post-operative tamponade, 1% myocardial infarction and 9% mediastinitis.

Out of 100 patients operated on, four cases of precocious endocarditis were observed post-operatively (4%), including one patient with preoperative endocarditis of a native valve. Only one case of precocious thrombosis of a mitral prosthesis, which was intermittently obstructive, was reported, following interruption of antiaggregant and anticoagulant treatment two months after surgery.

During the post-operative period, 21 early deaths occurred, representing a post-operative mortality rate of 19.8%, bringing the total number of deaths to 27 patients and a hospital mortality rate of 25.4%.

The causes of post-operative death were septic shock related to infectious pneumonitis in 10 cases (9.4%), infective endocarditis in 3 cases (3%), myocardial infarction in one patient, post-operative tamponade in six patients (5%) and cardiogenic shock in one patient (1%).

The following factors were predictive of mortality: administration of catecholamines (p = 0.042, OR = 85.8), pulmonary complications (p = 0.042, OR = 85.8), valve surgery performed in an emergency setting (p = 0.011, OR = 3.66), prolonged operating time (p = 0.016) and tamponade (p = 0.016, OR = 6.2).

The mean follow-up time from the last consultation was 54.5 months. We noted that dyspnea disappeared in 56 patients (84.8%) and improved in eight others (12.1%), moving from NHYA stage III to stage II.

Follow-up echocardiography revealed a good hemodynamic profile for the implanted bioprostheses in 90.9% of cases. Three patients had a stenosed bioprosthesis (5%) and two others had a leaky prosthesis (3%).

Only one late death was reported by the family, with no definite cause.

II. STRENGTHS AND LIMITATIONS OF OUR STUDY :

Our study is a multicentre study, carried out in three centres in Tunisia, thereby limiting selection bias. It is the largest Tunisian series in terms of the number of patients who have undergone valve replacement with a bioprosthesis.

There are few studies in the world, and none in Tunisia, that have dealt with the implantation of biological prostheses in patients under 65 years of age. Although our study was carried out before the revision of the ESC/EACTS 2021 recommendations [4], in which age was the determining factor for the choice of prosthesis, ten of our patients (9%), aged between 17 and 45 years, chose to have a bioprosthesis implanted because of poor compliance with therapy or for professional reasons.

Our study highlighted the low risk of short- and medium-term complications with biological prostheses, as well as their superior tolerability in the event of complications, in this case prosthesis obstruction, unlike mechanical prostheses, where no delay in diagnosis and management can be tolerated.

Our study has several limitations that need to be taken into account. The retrospective nature of this study and the small number of patients compared with worldwide series is one of its limitations and inevitably leads to a lack of power.

There is a selection bias, with some centres preferring to place bioprostheses only in elderly patients.

On the other hand, the relatively large number of patients lost to follow-up was an obstacle to analysing the follow-up of our patients using the Kaplan Meier gauge.

Finally, the concept of implanting cardiac bioprostheses in patients under 65 years of age was introduced late in our country compared with the West. As a result, a five-year follow-up does not allow us to study the long-term evolution of bioprostheses in the young population, which is another limitation of the study.

III. STRENGTHS AND LIMITATIONS OF THE MAIN FINDINGS IN THE LITERATURE :

Although there has been a significant change in valve surgical practice in the choice of prosthesis type over the last few decades, there have been few studies in the literature dealing independently with the subject of bioprostheses. Most of these studies tend to be comparative with mechanical prostheses, and between two groups that were not comparable, with older patients and higher operative risk in the biological prosthesis group.

Given the recent nature of the ESC/EACTS 2021 recommendations [4] (Appendix 2), which take into account the wishes of a well-informed patient when selecting a first-line prosthesis, it is clear that few studies are currently available concerning bioprostheses in subjects under 65 years of age.

In the absence of conclusive trials comparing the new generations of bioprostheses with the old models, the ESC 2021 recommendations concluded that there was only a C level of evidence for choosing the type of prosthesis. However, with the considerable development of new bioprostheses, the evidence in the literature suggests superior durability with less morbidity and mortality [4].

IV. THEORETICAL BACKGROUND :

1. HISTORY :

The first cardiac valve replacements were performed in the 1960s, with valve substitutes constantly evolving. Many prostheses have been invented since 1952 up to the present day (table XXIII). The main challenge was to have a prosthesis that was hemodynamically perfect with a minimum risk of complications and easy to implant surgically.

The ideal valve that is non-obstructive, continuous, does not degenerate, does not thrombose, does not alter the constituents of the blood, is easy to implant and is well tolerated by the patient still does not exist; however, many types of valve are coming closer and closer to achieving these objectives. Considerable progress has been made since the first heart valves were implanted, with a parallel improvement in hemodynamic profiles [9].

The first mechanical prostheses had balls inside. The 2eme generation of prostheses used discs. These two generations have now been abandoned and it is the new generation of mechanical prosthesis that is currently in use: the so-called double-fin prosthesis [3].

Table XXIII: Evolution of mechanical prostheses over time

1952	1965	End of 1960s	1969 1971 1982	1977	End of THE 70S
Dr. HUFNAGEL valve [10]	Dr. STARR's ball valve [11].	Beall disc valve [12]	Bjork swivel disc valve Shiley [13]	St Jude double winged valve [14].	Carbomedics double wing valve [15].
Quickly abandoned	Abandoned	Abandoned	Abandoned	Most used currently	Always used

Biological prostheses began to appear alongside implants using mechanical prostheses. In the early 1960s, experimentation with biological heart valves was initiated because of the post-operative thrombo-embolic complications observed with mechanical prostheses. Donald Ross used aortic homografts in 1962, followed by Barrat Boyes [16]. Subsequently, Jean-Paul Binet and Alain Carpentier, wishing at all costs to avoid the patient having to take anticoagulants for life, introduced a bioprosthesis of animal origin. In 1965, they implanted the first pig aortic heterografts treated with a mercury solution [17].

In 1968, Alain Carpentier improved the conditioning of these valves by using glutaraldehyde to ensure better tissue preservation and reduce the risk of immunological reactions, which lead to very early tissue deterioration [18]. The result was a biologically inert prosthesis with less tissue destruction.

In the following years, he decided to mount porcine heterografts on a frame to facilitate implantation, and gave them the name bioprosthesis. This became the most widely used biological prosthesis in the world, the only drawback being a limited lifespan [19]. However, with continuous technological innovation, the durability of bioprostheses has become increasingly superior and patients, who should be re-operated every 8 to 10 years, can live with them for 25 years or more.

In 1981, the first bovine pericardial bioprostheses were marketed [20].

Since then, numerous advances have made it possible to improve the flexibility of the framework, optimise tissue preservation, reduce stress on the cusps and reduce the thickness of the collars. Increasingly sophisticated anticalcic treatments have improved the durability of bioprostheses [21].

Their use has only increased over the last decade, far surpassing that of mechanics, thanks to the significant development of bioprostheses, which degenerate less quickly and become increasingly reliable.

2. VALVE SUBSTITUTES:

There are two types of heart valve prosthesis: so-called mechanical prostheses and biological prostheses. These are artificial valves consisting of a metal framework, which may or may not have a suture flange, inside which there are moving parts. Depending on the type of valve, mechanical or biological, these movable elements may be either metallic or based on biological material.

2.1. Types of biological prostheses :

There are three types of biological prostheses:

2.1.1. Autograft :

It consists of removing a valve from the patient's own heart and replacing it in another position. Only one technique is commonly used: the Ross procedure (developed by Donald Ross in 1967) [16]. It consists of removing the valve and the pulmonary artery and placing them in an aortic position. During the same period, Mr Ross proposed the Ross mitral or Ross II procedure, enabling the mitral valve to be replaced by the patient's own pulmonary valve [22].

2.1.2. Homografts:

Homografts are cryopreserved heart valves from human donors. They have perfect hemodynamics and degenerate slowly [23]. However, they are much less widely used due to their limited availability.

2.1.3. Heterografts or bioprostheses :

They are the most widely used. The main component of the prosthesis may be of porcine, bovine or equine origin. They are preserved with glutaraldehyde, which preserves their structure. There are three types of heterograft:

A. Bioprostheses with reinforcement or Stented :

They represent the majority of aortic valve substitutes. The pericardium used may be of bovine or porcine origin. The different bioprostheses with reinforcement are illustrated in table XXIV.

Table XXIV: Reinforced or stented bioprostheses

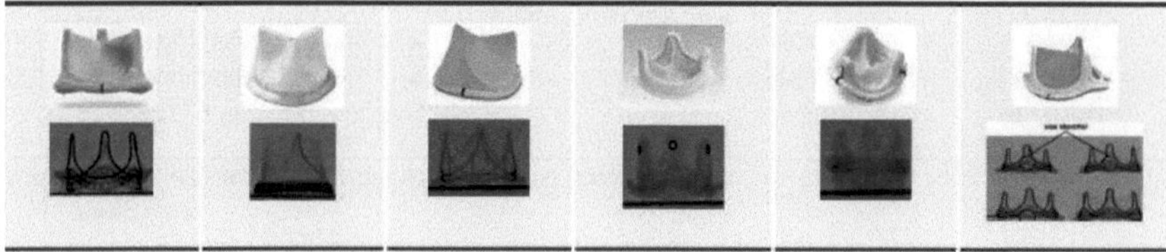

PERIMOUNT prosthesis (Edwards)	Prosthesis MITROFLOW [24]	TRIFECTA prosthesis [25]	HANCOCK prosthesis [26]	EPIC/ EPIC SUPRA prosthesis [27]	INSPIRIS prosthesis [28]
ý 3 independent cusps in bovine pericardium ý Metal frame	ý A single piece of bovine pericardium ý Flexible support	ý A single piece of bovine pericardium ý Titanium stent	ý 3 porcine pericardial cusps ý polymer stent	ý 3 porcine pericardial cusps ý polymer stent	ý Visible prosthesis stent for easy delivery ý Internal and short leaflets ý Flexible frame (extension capacity)
ý **Excellent**	ý Small	Accelerated	ý Can be	Supra-	Designed for

durability of the latest generation [29].	prosthesis ý Accelerated deterioration [30] ý No longer marketed	deterioration [31].	implanted in a supra-annular position ý Satisfactory long-term results [26].	annular implantation (modified collar) [27].	a future **valve-in-valve** [28].

B. Stentless bioprostheses:

They allow larger prosthetic rings to be implanted (table XXV).

However, implantation is difficult in the case of calcified or very small-calibre rings.

Table XXV: Stentless bioprostheses

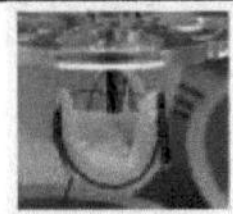	FREEDOM SOLO [32] prosthesis	■ Bovine pericardium	■　Supra-annular implantation ■　The most commonly used Stentless prosthesis [32].
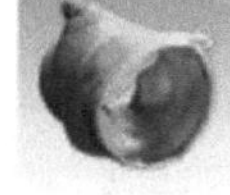	FREESTYLE prosthesis [33]	■　Explanted porcine aortic root ■　Piece of Dacron reinforcing the muscular sigmoid	■ Results comparable to other stent prostheses [33].

C. Sutureless bioprostheses:

These prostheses are intermediate in design between conventional and percutaneous prostheses (table XXVI). They are implanted intra-annularly under direct visual control, with 2/3 sutures or none at all. They therefore offer the possibility of a minimally invasive approach and a short clamping time.

Table XXVI: Sutureless bioprostheses

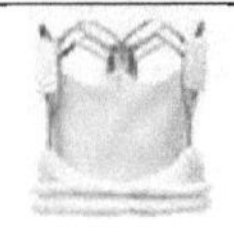	3F prosthesis Enable (ATS) [34]	■　The first sutureless prosthesis available ■　3 sheets in equine pericardium	■ Good hemodynamic characteristics ■ 18% rate of post-intervention pacemakers [35]
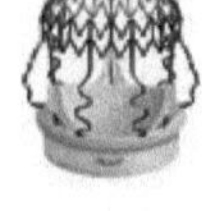	Perceval S (LinaNova) [36]	■　Structured on an alloy stent with bovine pericardium leaflets ■　Deployment by balloon expansion	■　Less para-prosthetic leakage ■　Good longevity ■　Pacemaker rate of 8% [36].
	Prosthesis S Intuity[37]	■ The Edwards surgical prosthesis meets the Sapien percutaneous prosthesis	■ Good hemodynamics ■Post-implantation pacemaker rate of 8%. [38]

2.1.4. **Choice of prosthesis :**

According to the latest recommendations of the European Society of Cardiology and the European Cardio-Thoracic Association, revised in 2021 [4], the first class I recommendation concerning the choice of type of prosthesis is in favour of the patient's wishes, whatever their age, after having been fully informed of the advantages and disadvantages of each type of valve (table XXVII).

Compared with previous recommendations, the emphasis is now on the importance of providing patients with complete, unbiased information during the selection process, rather than on their chronological age. The surgeon and cardiologist must explain the risks and benefits associated with each valve substitute to the patient in a precise and fair manner, so that the patient remains ultimately in control of the final decision regarding the choice of prosthesis. The patient must be given sufficient time to reflect, allowing him or her to seek a second opinion if necessary.

Table XXVII: ESC/EACTS 2021 recommendations for the choice of a bioprosthesis [4].		
Well-informed patient wishes	I	C
Impossibility of good quality anticoagulation (due to contraindication or high risk of bleeding or poor monitoring or lifestyle or professional activity)	I	C
Re-operation for a thrombosed mechanical prosthesis in a patient with poor coagulation control	I	C
Patients at low risk of valve redux surgery	IIa	C
Bioprosthesis should be considered for patients over 65 in the aortic position and over 70 in the mitral position, or those whose life expectancy is less than the presumed durability of the bioprosthesis. For patients aged 60-65 years who are to receive an aortic prosthesis, and patients aged between 65-70 years in the case of a mitral prosthesis, the 2 options (bioprosthesis or mechanical) are acceptable and the choice requires careful analysis of factors other than age.	IIa	C
Young woman wanting to become pregnant	IIa	C

V. POPULATION PROFILE :

1. Age :

The choice of prosthesis for valve replacement has changed significantly over the last few decades. Age is no longer the only determining factor in the selection of the type of prosthesis. The new recommendations concerning the choice of valve replacement are based on increasing the patient's life expectancy while improving their quality of life.

In a study comparing the results of mechanical and biological valve implantation in young subjects, Jones et al described a predominance of patients aged between 51 and 60 years, with an average age of 56 years [39].

Gabbrella et al [40] found that patients aged over 70 years were the most frequent.

Alexander Iribarne et al recommend that bioprosthesis implantation should be considered from the age of 50, and suggest that the final decision regarding the choice of prosthesis before the age of 65 remains a collective decision and must imperatively involve the patient [41].

In a study comparing bioprostheses with mechanical prostheses in a population aged under 50, Alperi A et al reported that the 15-year mortality rate was the same for both types of prosthesis [42]. In the latter study, neurological complications and post-operative bleeding were significantly lower in patients who had a bioprosthesis [42].

All these studies have concluded that bioprosthesis implantation at 50 years of age or over has no influence on 15-year survival.

The mean age of the population in our series was 68 ± 11.68 years [17-90], with 90% of patients aged over 60. This is in line with that described in most literature reviews. This can be explained by the fact that the study period for our series was conducted before the revision of the European recommendations. This age group tends to decrease more and more after 2021 in parallel with the advent of new biological valves characterised by their great longevity.

2. Gender :

The gender distribution of our patients showed a predominance of males (61%) compared with females (39%). This male predominance has been observed in the majority of international series. Douglas et al reported a male predominance of 64% in their series of 12569 patients who had undergone bioprosthesis implantation in the aortic position [43].

Although there is no direct correlation between the sex of patients and valve damage, recent studies of degenerative valve disease have shown that the female sex is becoming increasingly dominant in this population [44].

3. Professional activity :

The cumulative risk of hemorrhagic complications associated with the anticoagulant treatment required for valve replacement by mechanical prosthesis has become an increasingly important factor to take into account when considering the patient's quality of life. Several professions expose patients to the risk of trauma and injury, and therefore represent a constraint in the choice of the type of prosthesis.

The patient is therefore faced with a risk of bleeding increased by the anticoagulant treatment and the risk of long-term re-operation, which is becoming increasingly out of proportion with the longevity of bioprostheses. As a result, patients are increasingly reluctant to accept lifelong anticoagulant treatment and the associated constraints, particularly physical activity.

A study by M Ruel et al on the quality of life of patients who had a valve replacement between the ages of 18 and 50 showed that younger patients who had a bioprosthetic valve replacement, sparing them from anticoagulation, had a better quality of life than those who had a mechanical prosthesis[45].

In our series, three of our patients chose to have a bioprosthesis implanted because of their occupations that could cause bleeding: the first was a farmer, the second was a policeman and the last was a sports teacher.

4. Pregnancy and bioprosthesis :

In young women of childbearing age, pregnancy under anticoagulant treatment is particularly complex because of the risks to the fetus. The choice of a biological prosthesis is more judicious in order to avoid the teratogenic risks of anticoagulant treatment, which is also difficult to manage during pregnancy.

B R Badduke et al demonstrated in a study carried out at the University of British Columbia, Van couver, Canada that implantation of a bioprosthesis allowed a pregnancy without risk for the fetus and without an increase in maternal morbidity and mortality [46].

5. Impact on social life :

The quality of life of patients operated on with a biological valve is similar to that of non-operated subjects in the same age group. Unlike mechanical prostheses, the number of medical visits is lower, blood tests are less frequent and valve noises cannot be heard at a distance.

A study by Zhi-Nuan Hong et al in China of 103 patients who had undergone mechanical valve replacement showed that after one year of surgery, more than 10% of patients suffered from prosthesis noise-related stress, with a significantly reduced quality of life [47].

6. Cardiovascular risk factors :

6.1. Body mass index :

Analysis of BMI in our series showed that being overweight was associated with a significantly higher risk of death.

J Ernesto Molina et al have shown that obesity predisposes patients to surgical site complications [48]. Another study by Quoc-Sy Nguyen et al showed that BMI has an impact on the development of pulmonary infections due to altered respiratory mechanics [49].

In contrast, Vaduganathan et al concluded that patients with a BMI > 25 kg/m^2 have a lower risk of mortality than patients with a BMI < 18 kg/m2 [50].

6.2. Metabolic syndrome :

The main cardiovascular risk factors identified in our study were hypertension, smoking, dyslipidemia and diabetes. Metabolic syndrome, defined as a set of metabolic disturbances linked to insulin resistance and dyslipidemia, is an important predictor of degenerative valve sclerosis [51].

A recent study carried out in Quebec and published by Mathieu P, showed that these cardiovascular risk factors, being closely linked to the metabolic syndrome, are implicated in the progression of valve pathology [52]. In fact, these patients showed a more rapid progression of their valvular disease due to the pro-inflammatory effects directly activated and maintained by this syndrome within the valve [9].

Briand M et al have shown that metabolic syndrome is independently associated with rapid degeneration of bioprostheses and suggest, as a means of preventing this, the introduction of the necessary drugs to treat metabolic syndrome [53].

7. Associated pathologies:

7.1. Chronic renal failure (CRF):

According to the recommendations of the French National Authority for Health (HAS), CKD is defined as creatinine clearance of less than 60 ml/min/1.73m [54]. Renal insufficiency and phosphocalcium metabolism disorders are factors that favour calcification of bioprostheses and raise the question of their use in these situations due to the increased risk of structural degeneration [55].

However, in dialysis patients and in the absence of hyperparathyroidism, bioprostheses are preferred because they allow easier management of dialysis sessions from the point of view of anticoagulation.

Charles A Herzog et al demonstrated that no significant difference was found in survival rates between patients with renal failure at the hemodialysis stage who had a mechanical or biological prosthesis [43].

Zhibing et al reported a significantly lower rate of thrombo-embolic and hemorrhagic events in renal failure patients undergoing hemodialysis with a bioprosthesis compared with those with a mechanical prosthesis [56]. They also report a lower prosthesis-related mortality rate for bioprostheses [56].

In our series, six patients had chronic renal failure at the hemodialysis stage with a good hemodynamic profile of the bioprosthesis on remote ultrasound monitoring.

7.2. Rheumatic fever (RF):

Rheumatic fever is still common in developing countries and remains the main cause of acquired valve disease [57]. Rheumatic origin represents the 2eme cause in our series and 13 patients had a history of AAR from an early age.

8. Euroscore II :

Euroscore II is the most widely used risk score in Europe for patients undergoing cardiac surgery. It is used to estimate perioperative mortality before surgery by taking into account the patient's clinical and ultrasound data, in particular ejection fraction, creatinine clearance and certain factors such as pulmonary arterial pressure [58]. The higher the score, the higher the risk.

In the literature, the mean of this score varies between 0.8 and 15 according to the different series in subjects who have had valve replacement. A Brazilian series by Casalino R et al found a Euroscore II of 0.8 to 10 [59].

Czub et al report in their series a Euroscore II for patients proposed for aortic valve replacement of 3.2 ± 4, and for patients proposed for mitral valve replacement of 15.3 ± 19.4 [60].

For our series, the Euroscore II was 2.69% ± 1.17 [0.62% -7%].

VI. ETIOLOGIES :

1. Rheumatic diseases :

Although it has become rare in Western countries, AAR remains a public health problem in low-development countries. Prevention efforts, based on the treatment of pharyngeal infections, have significantly improved the management of this disease [57]. In our series, 39 of our patients (36.8%) had rheumatic valve disease.

2. Degenerative pathology :

They most often affect the elderly. Degenerative causes are currently the most common, dominated by aortic narrowing and mitral insufficiency. In industrialised countries, improved health conditions and an ageing population explain the change in the etiological distribution of acquired valve disease [61].

In our series, a predominance of degenerative valve disease was noted, affecting half of our patients (51.9%).

3. Infectious endocarditis :

It is secondary to infection of the endocardium by a bacterial micro-organism. It occurs more frequently in pre-existing valvulopathy when germs enter the bloodstream via a detectable portal of entry [62]. Eight of our patients (7.5%) had infective endocarditis.

4. Aortic bicuspid :

It is the most common congenital malformation [63]. Patients with aortic bicuspidism are predisposed to the development of infective endocarditis, stenosis and/or aortic leakage. The decision and timing of intervention for this condition depends on the size of the aorta, the function of the valve, and whether it is associated with other anomalies [64].

5. Barlow's disease :

It is one of the main causes of mitral insufficiency. It is characterised by an excess of valvular tissue leading to prolapse of one or both mitral leaflets [65].

VII. CLINICAL STUDY :

1. Circumstances of discovery :

Clinical manifestations are determined by the type of valve damage and the etiology involved. They can be either pauci-symptomatic or revealed by a complication.

2. Functional signs :

*2.1.*Dyspnea :

This is the most frequent symptom that leads patients to seek medical advice. It takes the form of dyspnea, which may appear gradually or suddenly, depending on the cause. It reflects the impact of left heart hyperpressure on the pulmonary circulation.

In the various worldwide series, NYHA stages III and IV predominated. Gabella and colleagues reported in their study that, at the time of surgery, 54% of their population were in NYHA stage III or IV [40].

In Great Britain, the study conducted by Alexander Iribarne et al found that 7.2% of patients had NYHA stage IV [41]. Stage II was noted in aortic disease.

The results of our series are in line with the literature. Dyspnea was the functional sign most frequently encountered in our study (80.1%). The majority of patients were at an advanced functional stage, with 45 patients at stage III (53.5%), while 39.5% of our study population had stage II dyspnoea.

2.2.Chest pain :

Chest pain may represent an angina attack or MI related to coronary embolism or coronary artery disease per se. In our series, chest pain was the 2eme reason for discovery in 37.7% of our patients.

2.3.Syncope and malaise:

They may be the only mode of expression and are seen in aortic valve disease. These syncopes and equivalents occur during effort and are related to the sudden fall in cardiac output and consequently cerebral output during excessive effort [66].

A study published by Goliasch G et al of 625 patients who had undergone aortic valve replacement surgery found a prevalence of 10.7% syncope with a significantly increased mortality rate [67].

In our series, 24 patients (22.6%) suffered syncope, eight of whom died, giving a mortality rate of 37%.

3. Physical signs :

3.1.Auscultatory abnormality :

The most important physical sign is an auscultatory abnormality. Its presence alone enables early diagnosis of valve damage before the onset of functional signs.

3.2.Signs of heart failure :

Left heart valve disease affects right ventricular function. Low flow and left-sided stasis initially result in acute lung redemas, and are then progressively supplemented by right-sided stasis causing peripheral redemas and ascites. Delayed diagnosis and surgical management are pejorative factors in the progression of heart failure [68].

In our series, 23.6% of our patients arrived at the surgical stage in heart failure, reflecting the advanced stage of their valve disease, with a rate of 19.6% in left heart failure and 4% in right heart failure.

3.3.Limb ischemia :

The symptoms include pain, coldness of the limb and sensory-motor signs. It is the result of peripheral embolism. Valvular damage was revealed in four of our patients (3.8%) by acute ischaemia of the limb.

3.4.Neurological deficit :

Neurological signs may be seen in particular during embolic accidents, such as motor deficit of a hemiparesis or hemiparesis. This clinical picture was seen in two patients in our series (1.8%).

In a study of 196 patients undergoing aortic valve replacement for calcific aortic narrowing, Messe et al reported a post-operative stroke and transient ischemic attack rate of 8% and a significantly high mortality rate [69].

4. Diagnostic means :
4.1.Chest X-ray :
It is a simple, rapid, easily accessible, inexpensive and low-radiation test, useful in the assessment of clinical cardiac abnormalities. It may be normal or show :
- An increase in the cardiothoracic ratio linked to cardiomegaly
- Signs of heart failure, in particular hilar overload
- Mitral silhouette due to progressive dilatation of the OG
- A protrusion of the aortic button

In our series, the chest X-ray was normal in 7 patients. Cardiomegaly was present in 49 patients (46.2%), reflecting the advanced stage of their valve disease, with hilar overload revealed in 22 cases (20.8%). Protrusion of the aortic button and mitral silhouette were observed in 79 and 10 cases respectively (74.5% and 9.4%).

4.2.Electrocardiogram :
It plays a key role in the assessment of valvular patients. It reveals rhythm and conduction disorders, ischaemic signs and also signs of ventricular hypertrophy.

Yeow L et al reported in their Mayo Clinic study of 323 patients who had undergone mitral valve replacement that the prevalence of AF was 30% [70].

AF was the rhythm disorder most frequently found in our patients (26.4%) and 11 patients had conductive disorders.

4.3.Echocardiography-doppler :
4.3.1. Trans-thoracic echocardiography :
TTE is the key test for diagnosing and monitoring heart valve disease. It is a rapid, non-invasive examination which allows the re-evaluation of valve structures and functions by providing multiple pieces of information:
- Confirm stenosis or valve regurgitation.
- Quantifying the severity of valve damage
- Identify the mechanism of valvular insufficiency and point to the etiology.
- To enable precise analysis of the morphological characteristics of the valvular and sub-valvular apparatus.
- To assess the impact on the heart chambers, overall cardiac function and pulmonary circulation.
- Monitoring the evolution of valvular disease and cardiac prosthesis after surgery.

4.3.2. Trans-resophageal echocardiography (TEE) :
TEE is an essential adjunct to TTE in many circumstances of valve pathology. Indications are dominated by endocarditis, the existence or absence of intra-atrial thrombus, per-operative interest, and re-evaluation of valve prostheses [71].

4.4.Cardiac scanner :
Cardiac CT has become an important tool in the study of native or prosthetic valve damage. Because of its specific ability to study calcifications, it is playing an increasingly important role in the study of heart valve disease, particularly degenerative heart valve disease. Because tissue thickening and the accumulation of calcifications limit the mobility of the valve leaflets, degenerative aortic narrowing lends itself to study by CT [72]. The latter can also be used to determine whether the aortic valve is bicuspid, with or without a raphe.

In the case of mitral narrowing, the frequent association with AF and a rapid, irregular heart rhythm makes the examination uninterpretable due to the kinetic artefacts associated with myocardial contractions. In the case of bioprostheses, calcifying degenerescence is visualised as in calcified aortic narrowing [73].

*4.5.*Preoperative coronary angiography :

When surgery is planned, coronary angiography is used to assess the state of the coronary network. The surgical procedure may be modified if there is associated coronary damage. However, this examination is invasive and not without risk.

5. Surgical treatment :

*5.1.*Goals :

5.1.1. Correction of valve function :

Any valvular disease causing significant repercussions must be corrected. Restoring correct valve function removes the mechanical obstruction to blood flow in the case of stenosis and prevents hypertrophy-dilatation of the heart chambers in the case of regurgitation.

The difficulty, in the case of a bioprosthesis, which may deteriorate at a later stage, lies in the surgical decision in relation to multiple valve lesions, one of which was initially assessed as moderate and which may subsequently increase, necessitating re-intervention. The surgeon is thus faced with a dilemma:

- Intervene at the stage of moderate damage, at the cost of extending the time of extracorporeal circulation and avoiding a second surgery.

- Respect the moderately damaged valve and reduce the operative risk, but expose the patient to subsequent redux surgery for further valve damage.

5.1.2. Prevention of complications :

The indication for valve surgery is based on an overall assessment of the consequences of the various types of valve damage and the risks of complications, in particular systemic embolisms, heart failure and sudden death.

*5.2.*Valvular gesture :

5.2.1. Mitral valve :

When the valve is so badly damaged, conservative surgery is not possible. This is the case for rheumatic conditions that are not amenable to valve repair because of the significant changes to the sub-valvular apparatus. Mitral valve replacement is performed with the aim of preserving the sub-valvular apparatus.

Muthialu et al concluded from their study of the impact of preserving the subvalvular apparatus during mitral valve replacement that this condition improves survival by preserving left ventricular function [74].

In our series, preservation of the posterior valve was the rule, with extensive rheumatic disease and endocarditis of the small valve being the only conditions requiring extensive resection of the entire valve.

5.2.2. Aortic valve :

Aortic valve replacement is the mainstay of treatment for symptomatic forms. Aortic valve resection is a simple procedure that can often be carried out without any problems. However, it is not without risk, particularly during intra-operative manipulation of valve calcifications.

5.2.3. Tricuspid valve :

Tricuspid surgery is dominated by conservative treatment because of the frequency of functional leaks concomitant with left heart valve disease. However, when the damage to the valve is too extensive, valve replacement is required.

In the tricuspid position, the implantation of mechanical prostheses is known to have a high rate of thrombosis and has led to the more frequent use of biological prostheses, which seem to degenerate less on the right side than on the left [75]. The difficulty in replacing the tricuspid valve is to avoid the conduction tissue. The most suitable technique is to use the remnants of the septal valve to suture the valve substitute, respecting the area of the anteroseptal commissure and the anterior part of the inner leaflet [76].

***5.3.*Combined gesture :**

The coexistence of valve disease, particularly degenerative valve disease, and coronary artery disease tends to increase with advancing patient age and the presence of co-morbidities. This association is increasingly detected in the absence of signs, thanks to pre-operative exploration of the coronary network in patients scheduled for valve surgery.

Combined surgery, previously considered too risky, has become safe and feasible. Advances in cardiac surgery in terms of surgical techniques and myocardial protection, as well as post-operative management, are constantly evolving and have improved the results of such major surgery.

In our series, eleven patients (10.4%) underwent combined surgery. Combined surgery was not associated with a significant increase in morbidity and mortality.

5.3.1. Coronary time :

After resection of the valve, distal coronary anastomoses are made first, especially for mitral valve replacement, as this requires dislocation of the creur, which cannot be performed once the prosthesis is in place [77]. Proximal anastomoses of any venous grafts are performed last after valve replacement under partial aortic clamping.

5.3.2. Valvular time :

The choice of valve substitutes may pose a problem in a valvular patient with a long life expectancy and in whom there is coronary damage for which surgical revascularisation is indicated.

A patient with a short life expectancy would probably not have time to deteriorate their bioprosthesis and would not be a candidate for redux surgery. However, for a patient with a longer life expectancy who is a candidate for valve replacement and simultaneous coronary bypass surgery, the decision as to which prosthesis to use is more difficult. The risk of degeneration of a bioprosthesis is increased in this case, and repeat surgery on a patient who has had coronary bypass surgery is associated with a higher operative mortality rate.

A metanalysis by Puvimanasinghe J et al, comparing 4274 patients who had undergone aortic valve surgery with a mechanical prosthesis and 9007 patients who had undergone valve replacement with a biological prosthesis, found that the use of a biological prosthesis combined with coronary bypass surgery did not increase morbidity or 10-year revision rates compared with patients who had undergone a mechanical prosthesis. They concluded that combined surgery with bioprosthesis could be proposed for younger subjects [77].

With the longevity of the new generations of biological prostheses and the "valve in valve" implantation technique, the choice of bioprosthesis is increasingly justified in these patients, whatever their age[78].

In our series, 11 patients (10.4%) underwent combined surgery. With a maximum follow-up of 5 years, the valve profile of these patients remained unchanged, with the exception of two patients who had moderately stenosing bioprostheses. Furthermore, in our study, combined surgery was not associated with an increase in morbidity and mortality.

***5.4.*Emergency valve surgery :**

Delayed management or acute endocarditis can lead to emergency surgery, increasing morbidity and mortality and jeopardising the patient's vital prognosis.

A. Iribarne et al, in their multicentre study, reported a rate of 18.1% of patients undergoing emergency surgery [41]. The rate of emergency valve surgery in our patients is close to that reported in the literature, i.e. 19.8%.

Emergency valve surgery is still associated with high morbidity and mortality. In a single-centre study published by Ibrahim et al of 346 patients who underwent valve replacement, mortality was significantly higher in the case of urgent surgery, with a mortality of 18.8% and an OR of 4.52 [79].

In our series, 12 patients (56%) who underwent emergency valve replacement died. Urgency was a predictive factor for mortality with a p of 0.011 and OR of 3.667.

6. Percutaneous treatment - valve-in-valve bioprosthesis:

The Valve-in-Valve technique for the degeneration of the surgical bioprosthesis appears to be an attractive alternative to valve surgery when a conventional re-intervention is deemed to have a very high surgical risk or even be potentially fatal. The procedure consists of introducing a percutaneous bioprosthesis via the femur and placing it within the old, degenerated bioprosthesis without recourse to extracorporeal circulation. Once the new prosthesis is in place, a balloon is used to deploy it and attach it to the old one.

The results of this technique appear to be encouraging. A recent study by Landes et al, including 330 patients who had either TAVI in TAV for percutaneous bioprosthesis degeneration or TAVI valve-in-valve for surgical bioprosthesis degeneration, found a similar complication rate and survival at 12 months between the two groups [80].

In a study by De Freitas Campos Guimaraes et al, involving 116 patients who had undergone valve-in-valve TAVI for deterioration of the aortic bioprosthesis, the short-term results were encouraging with a satisfactory success rate. Ultrasound follow-up at five years showed a stable transprosthetic gradient (less than 20%) and a low rate of degeneration estimated at 3% [78].

7. Intensive care unit management :

*7.1.*Length of stay :

The mean length of stay in intensive care in our series was 5 ± 6 days [1-58]. The total length of hospital stay was 12 ± 11 days [2-55].

Various studies have been carried out to assess the length of stay of patients undergoing valve surgery. The table below illustrates the average length of stay in intensive care and hospitalisation in a number of international series following implantation of cardiac bioprostheses.

Table XXVIII : Length of stay in resuscitation and hospitalisation compared with the literature

Study	Country	n	Length of stay in intensive care	Total length of stay
Ricardo Ferreira [81]	Portugal	196	3.3 [1-6.54]	7.7 [2-14]
KrishanRamsaransing[82]	Netherlands	110	1.4 [0.8-4]	8 [5-80]
Shreshta et al [83]	Germany	70	2 [1-4]	15.9 [5.9-26.8]
YesimGuner [84]	Turkey	52	1.9 [0.6-3.2]	7.6 [4.9-10.3]
Our series	Tunisia	106	5.14 [1-58]	12 [2-55]

The data found in the literature enabled us to situate ourselves in terms of the length of hospital stay for our patients. The length of stay in intensive care and the total length of hospitalisation appear to be high compared with the literature. This may be related to the frequency of post-operative pneumonitis and the need for NIV, given that many of our patients were known COPD patients.

*7.2.*Post-operative morbidity and mortality :

7.2.1. Morbidity:

7.2.1.1.   Complications unrelated to prostheses :
■ Bleeding complications :

Post-operative bleeding may be surgical in origin or related to post-CEC biological imbalance, given that CEC leads to consumption of coagulation factors, alteration of platelet function and activation of fibrinolysis [85]. Post-operative bleeding of a biological nature is corrected by optimising hemostasis with blood products and derivatives. In the case of surgical bleeding, it is important to know the indication for revision, which appears to increase hospital morbidity and mortality.

Kristensen et al, reported a three-fold increase in mortality in patients who were retreated for post-CEC surgical hemostasis [86].

The decision as to whether or not to repeat the operation is based on the recommendations of Kirklin and Barrat-Boyes, who, in addition to the amount of blood drained, take into account the kinetics of bleeding [87].

24 of our patients suffered post-operative haemorrhage, 16 of whom were taken back for surgery to check hemostasis.

■ Tamponade :

After cardiac surgery, and in particular after valve replacement, tamponade is the dreaded event for surgeons, significantly increasing morbidity and mortality.

Kurvin et al subdivide them into early tamponade before 24 hours and late tamponade after one day. Before 24 hours, the cause was uncontrolled or poorly controlled surgical bleeding, with hemodynamic instability leading to repeat surgery. Predisposing factors for late tamponade were female gender, pre-operative anticoagulation and low baseline haematocrit. Percutaneous drainage was possible in these cases [88,89].

In our series, 11 tamponades were identified, six of which occurred post-operatively, eight early and three late. Of these, 27% were on preoperative anti-coagulation for AF, 54% were on anti-platelet aggregation therapy and 10% were female, with an overall mortality rate of 5%.

■ Post-operative pneumonitis :

The occurrence of post-operative pulmonary infections has been described in various series. In the literature, the rate of pulmonary infections after valve surgery varies widely, from 2.8 to 23% [90,91].

Peng Xiao et al reported a pulmonary infection rate of 15.08%. This study found that the presence of a metabolic syndrome was a risk factor [92].

Riera M et al found an incidence of post-cardiac surgery pulmonary infections of 4% with predictive factors of LVEF less than 30%, chronic renal failure and the context of urgent surgery [93]. They also reported that among patients with post-operative infectious pneumonitis, mortality was 42% [93].

In our study, 52 patients (49%) presented with post-operative infectious pneumonitis with a good clinical-radiological evolution after adequate antibiotic therapy and respiratory kinesitherapy in 34 patients (34%).

Of our patients with post-operative pneumonia, 28% had undergone emergency surgery, 28% had COPD, 28% had had prolonged surgery, 26% had been intubated for more than 24 hours and 76% had stayed in intensive care for more than 48 hours.

Eighteen of the patients with infectious pneumopathy (34.6%) died of septic shock with a pulmonary onset. These figures are high compared with the literature. This is probably due to the aseptic conditions imposed by Tunisian health facilities, despite the respiratory preparation of bronchial patients and the targeted treatment of pre-operative pulmonary infections aimed at shortening the hospital stay and avoiding these serious pulmonary complications.

■ Post-operative rhythm disorders :

18 patients (18%) who were in sinus rhythm before valve replacement went into AF post-operatively. These patients retained a permanent arrhythmia requiring long-term anticoagulant treatment. Conversely, chronic AF was reduced spontaneously or by cardioversion during weaning from bypass surgery in 6 patients. However, this reduction was transient and the rhythm returned to fibrillation.

Filardo G et al reported a rate of de novo AF following valve surgery of 37%. The risk factors for the onset of AF were advanced age and association with coronary bypass surgery [94].

Kalra R et al found a 50% incidence of de novo AF, 69% of which occurred in patients who had a bioprosthesis compared with 30.9% for mechanical valves. Hospital mortality was significantly higher in these patients [95].

Bjorn MD et al reported an incidence of de novo AF of 42.6%. Valve replacements with bioprostheses were associated with de novo AF in 50% of cases, whereas mechanical prostheses were associated with de novo AF in 25% of cases [96]. For Bjorn et al, the rate of reversibility of de novo AF was 10% for all patients, with 20% for bioprostheses and no reversibility was found for mechanical prostheses. New cases of AF appeared in patients with mechanical prostheses during remote follow-up [96].

This high rate of de novo AF in bioprosthesis wearers was explained by the association with older age in the two previous studies, compared with mechanical prostheses. For Bjorn et al, the average age of bioprosthesis implantation was 76, compared with 60 for mechanical prostheses. Advanced age was a consistent risk factor for the development of de novo AF in the majority of studies [94-96].

In our series, mortality was 11% in patients with de novo AF, of whom four (22.5%) had associated coronary surgery and 61% were aged over 70.

■ Conduction disorders :

The risk of developing conductive disorders after valve surgery varies according to the series, from 7 to 15% [97].

Ferrari et al reported an incidence of post-operative conductive disorders of 17%. The risk factors were age over 60, AF, pre-operative beta-blocker use, bioprosthesis implantation, mitral valve surgery and chronic renal failure [98].

Viles-Gonzalez et al found an incidence of AVB of 23.7% in 290 patients undergoing mitral valve replacement. Predictive factors were age, prosthesis size and prolonged duration of bypass surgery [99].

Elahi et al have shown that implantation of a small bioprosthesis is associated with a relatively high rate of permanent AVB due to the incongruence of its framework, even at a small size, in a relatively narrow and calcified ring, inducing lesions of the conduction tissue [100].

In our series, seven patients (7%) who had no pre-operative conduction problems developed a post-operative 3rd degree BAV, two of whom required a permanent pacemaker. Of these patients, 55% were over 65 years of age, 11% were initially in AF and 22% had undergone mitral valve surgery compared with 78% who had undergone aortic valve surgery.

■ Post-operative MI :

The literature review showed a rate of post-operative MI of 0.7 to 11.8% after combined surgery [101]. In our series, this occurred in a single patient who had coronary artery bypass grafting (CABG) concomitant with valve replacement.

7.2.1.1. Complications associated with prostheses :

■ Early endocarditis :

Although rare, infective endocarditis is the most serious complication of valve replacement. Early endocarditis occurs within 60 days of the operation and is due to peri-operative contamination. Diagnosis is based on the results of blood cultures and echocardiography, which allow a precise assessment of lesions and prosthetic dysfunction [102].

The clinical profile consists of a febrile picture, which must be distinguished from respiratory infections; septic shock sometimes develops. Infection of biological prostheses involves the valve tissue.

The mechanism by which endocarditis develops on biological valves is explained by bacterial grafting onto the cusps of the bioprostheses. This phenomenon is minimal during the first few years following implantation of the bioprosthesis. With progressive degeneration of the biological tissue, structural lesions begin to develop, favouring bacterial grafting and significantly increasing the rate of infective endocarditis [103].

In a series of 310 patients (155 with bioprosthesis and 155 with mechanical prosthesis), Stassano et al reported a lower incidence of infective endocarditis in subjects with bioprosthesis compared with those with mechanical prosthesis [104].

Prosthetic endocarditis continues to have a poor prognosis, particularly at the stage of evolving complications such as abscesses, pseudoaneurysm and hemodynamic failure.

In our study, four cases of precocious endocarditis were observed post-operatively (4%) in two patients known to be diabetic and two admitted with heart failure, one of whom had pre-operative endocarditis on a native valve. One patient had a favourable outcome with appropriate antibiotic therapy. The other three patients required urgent revision surgery for refractory heart failure.

■ Prosthesis thrombosis :

They are less serious with biological prostheses and are less obvious. It is often a non-obstructive thrombosis. This is favoured by hemodynamic and hemostatic factors such as poor compliance with therapy or inadequate anticoagulant treatment in the case of AF on a bioprosthesis.

Thrombosis of biological prostheses generally has a better immediate prognosis than thrombosis of mechanical prostheses, which are often obstructive and have a high mortality rate [105]. Bioprosthesis thrombosis usually progresses favourably after intensification of anticoagulant therapy in association with antiplatelet agents [106].

Egbe et al published a study demonstrating the efficacy of Warfarin for bioprosthesis thrombosis. The trans-prosthetic gradient improved in 83% of patients after ± 11 months of effective anticoagulation [105].

In our series, we noted a single intermittent precocious obstructive thrombosis (1%) in a mitral prosthesis following the interruption of antiaggregant and anticoagulant treatment by the patient two months before surgery. The patient made the same choice of prosthesis before undergoing a second mitral valve operation with simple post-operative follow-up.

■ Degeneration of bioprostheses :

The degenerescence of biological prostheses, which was long considered to be a major drawback limiting their implantation, particularly in young patients, has tended to diminish over the years with the constant progress of bioprostheses, which have become increasingly durable. This gradual deterioration in bioprostheses is the result of several factors, which can be divided into two groups:

■ *Factors related to the prosthesis eiie-тёте :*

Such as its architecture and the chemical treatment of biological tissues [107].

- Patient factors :

In particular, the patient's age and the site where the prosthesis is implanted. Calcification of biological tissue is more rapid in younger patients. This progression towards calcification involves lipid metabolism, immunological reactions and disorders of phosphocalcium metabolism [108].

Bioprostheses degenerate more in the mitral position than in the aortic position, due to the greater structural damage of mechanical origin during mitral closure. For this reason, many surgeons have lowered the age limit for implantation of a bioprosthesis in the aortic position [109].

Guenzingeret al, found a much lower rate of prosthetic degeneration for the new bioprosthesis models in the long term, less than 10% at 10 years and less than 25% at 20 years, compared with an estimated rate of more than 40% at 20 years for the older generations [110].

Prosthetic degeneration in the mitral position has a more striking symptomatology with the progressive reappearance of dyspnoea and right signs compared with the aortic position where symptoms may be absent despite impaired left ventricular function [111].

A recent study by Raghav et al to assess the durability of the Edwards Magna Ease valve, by testing it in vitro at a stress equivalent to 25 years of life, found satisfactory results with preserved hemodynamics and structure, i.e. an estimated durability of more than 25 years [112].

In our series, no cases of degenerescence were found, given the five-year delay in our study.

■ Prosthetic insertion :

After valve replacement, small para-prosthetic leaks may occur before the annulus has completely healed. Disinsertion of the prosthesis may be the result of endocarditis due to suture loosening, or may be secondary to suturing over fragile tissue in an elderly patient or calcification of the annulus [113,114]. Exceptionally, it may be due to fracture of a cusp of a calcified bioprosthesis [115].

There was no evidence of reinsertion in any of our patients. However, two patients had a grade 1 to 2 central prosthetic leak on ultrasound examination.

7.2.2. Mortality :

In the literature, the rate of early death after valve surgery has improved markedly from ±30% in the 1990s to ±10% in recent years, independent of patient age and comorbidities [116].

In Suri's series, mean overall mortality fell progressively from 17% in 1993 to 9% in 2011, despite an increase in risk factors in the population studied [117].

In our series, we have noted :

-   6 per-operative deaths due to cardiopulmonary arrest (5.6%).

-   21 cases of post-operative death due to septic shock, ten related to infectious pneumonitis, six to tamponade, three to infective endocarditis, one to cardiogenic shock and one to myocardial infarction.

We identified the following factors as being predictive of mortality: valve surgery performed in an emergency setting, prolonged operating times and post-operative pulmonary infections.

We also found that post-operative mortality was higher in overweight patients and those with aortic insufficiency. Total mortality was equally high in men and women.

These factors are consistent with the literature, and mortality does not appear to be linked to complications of bioprostheses. A biological prosthesis may thrombose and become infected, but to a lesser degree than a mechanical prosthesis. The clinical symptoms associated with bioprosthesis complications are usually well tolerated, and management may be limited to intensification of medical treatment.

The morbidity and mortality associated with valve surgery is not negligible, particularly if it is carried out in an emergency situation and is associated with prolonged operating times. Added to this is the high frequency of post-operative pneumopathy and the significant costs that this entails. It is therefore essential to take steps to reduce the incidence of major cardiac events, as well as non-cardiac events, by limiting the complications of prosthetic heart valves and anticoagulant treatment.

This has been made possible by the increased longevity of bioprostheses, combined with constant advances in percutaneous techniques, which offer an excellent alternative when surgical bioprostheses degenerate.

6 CONCLUSIONS

Cardiac valve replacements, which began in 1960 with mitral valve replacement, have undergone several revolutions, starting with the invention of the ball prosthesis with anticoagulant treatment that had to be taken for life, moving on to the introduction of an animal bioprosthesis replacing steel with pig valves, and culminating in the advent of percutaneous techniques and the introduction of a bioprosthesis within an old degenerated bioprosthesis.

We conducted a retrospective, descriptive, multicentre, cross-sectional study in the cardiovascular surgery departments of the Abderrahmen Mami University Hospital in Ariana, the Habib Bourguiba University Hospital in Sfax, and the Tunis Military Hospital, between September 2017 and December 2021. We collected 106 patients operated on for valve replacement with a bioprosthesis.

The aims of our work were to describe the clinical and evolutionary profile of patients who had undergone valve replacement with a biological prosthesis and to determine the factors predictive of post-operative morbidity and mortality.

The patients included are those who have had one or more bioprostheses in any position (mitral, aortic and/or tricuspid), whether or not associated with coronary surgery.

Clinical and epidemiological data were recorded at inclusion, as well as intra- and post-operative complications, survival and functional status for each patient. A statistical study was performed including:

- A uni-variate study of immediate pre-, intra- and post-operative outcomes in relation to morbidity and mortality.

- A multivariate study of factors predictive of per- and post-operative morbidity and mortality.

In our study, the average age of patients was 68, with an estimated 9% aged between 17 and 45. The proportion of men (n=64) was greater than that of women (n=42), with a sex ratio of 1.52.

Arterial hypertension was the main cardiovascular risk factor. It was found in 59 patients (55.7%). The other risk factors were: smoking (41.5%), diabetes (29.2%), dyslipidemia (23.6%) and obesity (27.1%).

Thirteen patients had a history of rheumatic fever (12.3%). Other associated pathologies were chronic obstructive pulmonary disease (41.5%), associated coronary artery disease (20.7%), renal insufficiency (6.6%) and drug addiction (0.9%).

Seven patients had a history of prior cardiac surgery (6.6%). Mitral commissurotomy was performed in two patients (1.9%). Three patients had a history of mitral valve replacement (2.8%) and three had a history of aortic valve replacement (2.8%).

In our series, degenerative valve disease was predominant. It was present in 55 patients (51.90%), followed by rheumatic pathology in 39 patients (36.8%), then infective endocarditis in eight patients (7.5%).

The other etiologies were: aortic bicuspidity (1.9%), Barlow's disease (2.8%), ischemic etiology (1.9%) and systemic lupus erythematosus (0.9%).

The clinical presentation was polymorphous. In our series, the most frequent functional sign was dyspnoea, present in 85 patients (80.2%), with stage III predominating at 53.3%, followed by stage II at 39.5%.

Other signs included chest pain (37.7%), palpitations (36.8%) and a syncopal episode (22.6%). Occasionally, valvulopathy was diagnosed as a complication: limb ischemia (3.8%), cerebrovascular accident (1.8%). Elsewhere, it was identified accidentally in asymptomatic patients (3.8%) and the diagnosis was made during an echocardiography performed for another reason.

Twenty-five patients had heart failure (23.5%). An auscultatory abnormality was detected at the mitral site in 26 patients (24.5%) and at the aortic site in 86 patients (81.1%).

Echocardiography, considered to be the reference examination for diagnosing valvulopathy and determining its characteristics, has made it possible to evaluate left and right ventricular function, assess the impact on the pulmonary circulation and monitor the evolution of valvulopathy and the cardiac prosthesis after surgery.

The mean LV ejection fraction of the patients was 61% ± 0.08. The mean pulmonary artery pressure was 36.4% ± 13.35, with severe pre-operative PAH in 24 patients (22.4%). The left ventricle was dilated in 19 patients (17.9%), while right ventricular dilatation was found in seven patients (6.6%).

Aortic valve disease predominated in 85 patients (80.1%). Mitral valve disease was observed in 22 cases (20.7%). Tricuspid involvement was described in 10 patients (9.4%). The majority of patients had single valve disease (84.9%). Sixteen patients had double valve disease (15%) and no patient had triple valve disease.

Preoperative coronary angiography was used to diagnose significant coronary lesions in 21 patients, 11 of whom (10.4%) underwent coronary bypass surgery at the same time as valve surgery.

The mean predicted patient mortality according to Euroscore II was 2.69% ± 1.17.

23 patients underwent emergency surgery (21.7%). The circumstances justifying emergency surgery were numerous and generally related to a complication. These were either cardiac failure, following a syncopal episode or embolic accident, or related to prosthesis dysfunction.

All patients underwent bypass surgery with aortic clamping. Aortic valve replacement was performed in the majority of patients (81%), mitral valve replacement was performed in 26 patients (24.5%), while tricuspid valve replacement was performed in 10 patients (9.4%).

The mean duration of bypass surgery was 100.83 ± 33 minutes and the mean duration of aortic clamping was 74.94 ± 41.45 minutes.

Vasoactive drugs were not used at the end of the bypass in 16 patients (15%). On the other hand, 53 patients required low-dose catecholamines at the end of the bypass procedure (50%), while 37 patients (35%) required high-dose catecholamines.

Of the 106 patients operated on, 9 (8.4%) developed conduction problems intraoperatively. Six intra-operative deaths were reported as a result of an impossible exit from extracorporeal circulation (5.6%).

The average extubation time was 11 ± 33 hours.

The average length of stay in intensive care was 5 ± 6 days. Total hospital stay was 12 ± 11 days.

29 patients were weaned off vasoactive drugs in the operating theatre (27%). Weaning of patients was easy with low doses of catecholamines in 40.6% of cases and difficult in 23.6% of cases.

Out of 100 patients operated on, 24 developed post-operative bleeding, 16 of whom (16%) underwent repeat surgery to check hemostasis.

18 patients (18%) who were in sinus rhythm before the operation went into atrial fibrillation post-operatively, and seven patients (7%) who had no conductive problems pre-operatively developed atrioventricular block (AVB) 3eme post-operatively. Two patients were fitted with devices for definitive 3eme degree AVB, while the conductive disorders regressed in the other

five.

Post-operatively, we noted 54% of infectious pneumopathies, 17% of acute lung injury, 11% of post-operative tamponade, 1% of myocardial infarction and 9% of mediastinitis.

Out of 100 patients operated on, four cases of precocious endocarditis were observed post-operatively (4%), including one patient with pre-operative endocarditis on a native valve.

We noted a single intermittent obstructive thrombosis on a mitral prosthesis following interruption of antiaggregant and anticoagulant treatment after two months of surgery.

In our series, 21 early deaths occurred during the post-operative period, giving a post-operative mortality rate of 19.8%, bringing the total number of deaths to 27 patients and a hospital mortality rate of 25.4%.

The causes of post-operative death were septic shock related to infectious pneumonitis in 10 cases (9.4%), infective endocarditis in 3 cases (3%), myocardial infarction in one patient, post-operative tamponade in six patients (5%) and cardiogenic shock in one patient (1%).

Of the 100 patients who survived the hospital period, 66% were contacted and clinically monitored. The mean follow-up time from the last consultation was 54.5 months (6 months - 70 months).

We found that dyspnoea disappeared in 56 patients (84.8%) and improved in eight others (12.1%), moving from NHYA stage III to stage II.

Patients who had syncope pre-operatively did not have a syncopal episode after the operation. Two patients (3%) who had cardiac decompensation pre-operatively retained signs of heart failure.

All patients contacted were monitored by echocardiography. The time between surgery and echocardiography ranged from six to 66 months.

Follow-up echocardiography revealed a good hemodynamic profile for the implanted bioprostheses in 90.9% of cases. Four patients had a stenosed bioprosthesis (6%) and two others had a leaky prosthesis (3%).

We noted an improvement in pulmonary arterial hypertension in 24 patients (36.6%), three of whom had severe pre-operative PAH ranging from 65 to 80 mmHg and rising to between 25 and 40.

The EF at control was 52 ± 0.08%.

34 patients (51.5%) still had LVH on ultrasound examination, while 11 patients (16.6%) who had pre-operative LVH did not.

Only one late death was reported by the family, with no definite cause.

The following factors were predictive of mortality: administration of high-dose catecholamines with a p of 0.042 and an OR of 85.8, pulmonary complications with a p of 0.042 and an OR of 85.8, valve surgery performed in an emergency setting (p= 0.011; OR= 3.66), prolonged operating time (p= 0.016) and tamponade (p=0.016; OR= 6.2).

Our work has demonstrated the many advantages of bioprostheses over mechanical prostheses, in particular by offering patients receiving a biological valve a quality of life comparable to that of non-operated subjects. The risk of reoperation is no longer an issue for patients when it comes to selecting a bioprosthesis, given the increased longevity associated with the constant advances in percutaneous techniques.

A biological prosthesis can become thrombosed and infected, but this is less serious than with a mechanical prosthesis. The clinical picture is often well tolerated, and management may be limited to optimising medical treatment.

The main limitation of our work remains its retrospective nature and the timing of the study, which coincided with the period preceding the revision of the latest recommendations. In addition, our study is a first step towards carrying out similar work involving a younger population with a larger workforce. This will make it possible to better study the long-term evolution of cardiac bioprostheses and to have more data aimed at standardisation in the selection of the type of prosthesis in the various cardiovascular surgery departments in Tunisia.

REFERENCES

1. Siddiqui RF, Abraham JR, Butany J. Bioprosthetic heart valves: modes of failure. Histopathology. 2009 Aug;55(2):135-44.

2. Ribeiro GS, Tartof SY, Oliveira DS, Guedes AS, Reis MG, Riley LW, et al. Surgery for valvular heart disease: a population-based study in a Brazilian urban center.PLoS One. 2012 May;7(5):e37855.

3. Russo M, Taramasso M, Guidotti A, Pozzoli A, Nietilspach F, Von Segesser L, et al. The evolution of surgical valves. Cardiovasc Med. 2017 Dec;20(12):285-92.

4. Vahanian A, Beyersdorf F, Praz F, Milojevic M, Baldus S, Bauersachs J, et al. 2021 ESC/EACTS guidelines for the management of valvular heart disease. Eur Heart J. 2022 Feb;43(7):561-632.

5. Bartus K, Litwinowicz R, Sadowski J, Filip G, Kowalewski M, Suwalski P, et al. Bioprosthetic or mechanical heart valves: prosthesis choice for borderline patients?Results from 9,616 cases recorded in Polish national cardiac surgery registry. J Thorac Dis. 2020 Oct;12(10):5869-78.

6. Jougon J, Delcambre F, Velly JF. Anterior surgical approaches to the thorax. EMC - Techniques chirurgicales - Thorax 2006;1(1):1-20 [Article 42-210]

7. Pezzella AT, Effler DB, Levy IE. Operative approaches to the left atrium and mitral valve apparatus. Tex Heart Inst J. 1983 Jun;10(2):119-23.

8. Anger J, Dantas DC, Arnoni RT, Farsky PS. A new classification of post-sternotomy dehiscence. Rev Bras Cir Cardiovasc. 2015 Jan;30(1):114-8.

9. Kueri SA, Kari F, Ayala Fuentes R, Sievers HH, Beyersdorf F, Bothe W. The use of biological heart valves. Dtsch Arztebl Int. 2019 Jun;116(25):423-30.

10. Butany J, Ahluwalia MS, Fayet C, Munroe C, Blit P, Ahn C. Hufnagel valve: the first prosthetic mechanical valve. Cardiovasc Pathol. 2002 Nov;11(6):351-3.

11. Starr A. The starr-edwards valve. J Am Coll Cardiol. 1985 Oct;6(4):899-903.

12. Jassal DS, Miller R, Johnstone DE, Hirsch G. Beall mitral valve. Can J Cardiol. 2003 Nov;19(12):1445.

13. Bjork VO, Lindblom D. The monostrut bjork-shiley heart valve. J Am Coll Cardiol. 1985 Nov;6(5):1142-8.

14. Czer LS, Chaux A, Matloff JM, DeRobertis MA, Nessim SA, Scarlata D, et al. Ten-year experience with the St. Jude medical valve for primary valve replacement. J Thorac Cardiovasc Surg. 1990 Jul;100(1):44-54.

15. Copeland JG. TheCarboMedics prosthetic heart valve: a second generation bileaflet prosthesis. Semin Thorac Cardiovasc Surg. 1996 Jul;8(3):237-41.

16. Ross DN. Homograft replacement of the aortic valve. Lancet. 1962 Sep;2(7254):487.

17. O'Brien MF, Clareborough JK. Heterograft aortic-valve replacement. Lancet. 1967 Apr;1(7496):929-30.

18. Carpentier A, Lemaigre G, Robert L, Carpentier S, Dubost C. Biological factors affecting long-term results of valvular heterografts. J Thorac Cardiovasc Surg. 1969 Oct;58(4):467-83.

19. Chaikof EL. The development of prosthetic heart valveslessons in form and function. N Engl J Med. 2007 Oct;357(14):1368-71.

20. Ionescu MI, Pakrashi BC, Holden MP, Mary DA, Wooler GH. Results of aortic valve replacement with frame-supported fascia lata and pericardial grafts. J Thorac Cardiovasc Surg. 1972 Sep;64(3):340-53.

21. Gott JP, Girardot MN, Girardot JM, Hall JD, Whitlark JD, Horsley WS, et al. Refinement of the alpha aminooleic acid bioprosthetic valve anticalcification technique. Ann Thorac Surg.

1997 Jul;64(1):50-8.

22. Athanasiou T, Cherian A, Ross D. The ross II procedure: pulmonary autograft in the mitral position. Ann Thorac Surg. 2004 Oct;78(4):1489-95.

23. Nappi F, Al Attar N, Spadaccio C, Chello M, Lusini M, Acar C. Aortic valve homograft: 10year experience. Surg Technol Int. 2014 Mar;24:265-72.

24. Bleiziffer S, Eichinger WB, Hettich IM, Ruzicka D, Badiu CC, Guenzinger R, et al. Hemodynamic characterization of the sorin mitroflow pericardial bioprosthesis at rest and exercise. J Heart Valve Dis. 2009 Jan;18(1):95-100.

25. Malvindi PG, Kattach H, Luthra S, Ohri S. Modes of failure of trifecta aortic valve prosthesis. Interact Cardiovasc Thorac Surg. 2022 Jul;35(2): ivac086.

26. Fann JI, Miller DC. Porcine valves: hancock and carpentier-edwards aortic prostheses. Semin Thorac Cardiovasc Surg. 1996 Jul;8(3):259-68.

27. Maitland A, Hirsch GM, Pascoe EA. Hemodynamic performance of the St. Jude medical epic supra aortic stented valve. J Heart Valve Dis. 2011 May;20(3):327-31.

28. Tamagnini G, Bourguignon T, Rega F, Verbrugghe P, Lamberigts M, Langenaeken T, et al. Device profile of the inspiris resilia valve for aortic valve replacement: overview of its safety and efficacy. Expert Rev Med Devices. 2021 Mar;18(3):239-24.

29. Bourguignon T, Bouquiaux Stablo AL, Candolfi P, Mirza A, Loardi C, May MA, et al. Very long-term outcomes of the carpentier-edwards perimount valve in aortic position. Ann Thorac Surg. 2015 Mar;99(3):831-7.

30. Senage T, Le Tourneau T, Foucher Y, Pattier S, Cueff C, Michel M, et al. Early structural valve deterioration of mitroflow aortic bioprosthesis: mode, incidence, and impact on outcome in a large cohort of patients. Circulation. 2014 Dec;130(23):2012-20.

31. Fukuhara S, Shiomi S, Yang B, Kim K, Bolling SF, Haft J, et al. Early structural valve degeneration of trifecta bioprosthesis. Ann Thorac Surg. 2020 Mar;109(3):720-7.

32. Wollersheim LW, Li WW, Bouma BJ, Repossini A, Van Der Meulen J, De Mol BA. Aortic valve replacement with the stentless freedom solo bioprosthesis: a systematic review. Ann Thorac Surg. 2015 Oct;100(4):1496-504.

33. Ennker J, Meilwes M, PonsKuehnemann J, Niemann B, Grieshaber P, Ennker IC, et al. Freestyle stentless bioprosthesis for aortic valve therapy: 17-year clinical results. Asian Cardiovasc Thorac Ann. 2016 Nov;24(9):868-74.

34. Martens S, Sadowski J, Eckstein FS, Bartus K, Kapelak B, Sievers HH, et al. Clinical experience with the ATS 3f Enable® sutureless bioprosthesis. Eur J Cardiothorac Surg. 2011 Sep;40(3):749-55.

35. Aymard T, Kadner A, Walpoth N, Gober V, Englberger L, Stalder M, et al. Clinical experience with the second-generation 3f enable sutureless aortic valve prosthesis. J Thorac Cardiovasc Surg. 2010 Aug;140(2):313-6.

36. Dokollari A, Ramlawi B, Torregrossa G, Sa MP, Sicouri S, Prifti E, et al. Benefits and pitfalls of the perceval sutureless bioprosthesis. Front Cardiovasc Med. 2022 Jan;8:1-11.

37. Glauber M, Miceli A, Di Bacco L. Sutureless and rapid deployment valves: implantation technique from A to Z-the INTUITY elite valve. Ann Cardiothorac Surg. 2020 Sep;9(5):417-23.

38. Arribas Leal JM, Rivera Caravaca JM, Aranda Domene R, Moreno Moreno JA, Espinosa Garcia D, Jimenez Aceituna A, et al. Mid-term outcomes of rapid deployment aortic prostheses in patients with small aortic annulus. Interact Cardiovasc Thorac Surg. 2021 Oct;33(5):695-701.

39. Jones EL, Weintraub WS, Craver JM, Guyton RA, Cohen CL, Corrigan VE, et al. Ten-year

experience with the porcine bioprosthetic valve: interrelationship of valve survival and patient survival in 1,050 valve replacements. Ann Thorac Surg. 1990 Mar;49(3):370-83.

40. Rodriguez Gabella T, Voisine P, Dagenais F, Mohammadi S, Perron J, Dumont E, et al. Long-term outcomes following surgical aortic bioprosthesis implantation. J Am Coll Cardiol. 2018 Apr;71(13):1401-12.

41. Iribarne A, Leavitt BJ, Robich MP, Sardella GL, Gelb DJ, Baribeau YR, et al. Tissue versus mechanical aortic valve replacement in younger patients: a multicenter analysis. J Thorac Cardiovasc Surg. 2019 Dec;158(6):1529-38.

42. Alperi A, Hernandez Vaquero D, Pascual I, Diaz R, Silva I, AlvarezCabo R, et al. Aortic valve replacement in young patients: should the biological prosthesis be recommended over the mechanical? Ann Transl Med. 2018 May;6(10):183.

43. Johnston DR, Soltesz EG, Vakil N, Rajeswaran J, Roselli EE, Sabik JF, et al. Long-term durability of bioprosthetic aortic valves: implications from 12,569 implants. Ann Thorac Surg. 2015 Apr;99(4):1239-47.

44. He S, Deng H, Jiang J, Liu F, Liao H, Xue Y, et al. The evolving epidemiology of elderly with degenerative valvular heart disease: the Guangzhou (China) heart study. Biomed Res Int. 2021 Apr;2021:1-8.

45. Ruel M, Kulik A, Lam BK, Rubens FD, Hendry PJ, Masters RG, et al. Long-term outcomes of valve replacement with modern prostheses in young adults. Eur J Cardiothorac Surg. 2005 Mar;27(3):425-33

46. Badduke BR, Jamieson WR, Miyagishima RT, Munro AI, Gerein AN, MacNab J, et al. Pregnancy and childbearing in a population with biologic valvular prostheses. J Thorac Cardiovasc Surg. 1991 Aug;102(2):179-86.

47. Hong ZN, Huang JS, Huang LQ, Cao H, Chen Q. The effect of valve noise on the quality of life of patients after mechanical mitral valve replacement in a Chinese population. J Cardiothorac Surg. 2019 Jul;14(1):137-43.

48. Molina JE, Lew RL, Hyland KJ. Postoperative sternal dehiscence in obese patients: incidence and prevention. Ann Thorac Surg. 2004 Sep;78(3):912-7.

49. Nguyen QS, Choi C, Khoche S. Obesity and its implications for cardiac surgery patients. Int Anesthesiol Clin. 2020 Oct;58(3):34-40.

50. Vaduganathan M, Lee R, Beckham AJ, Andrei AC, Lapin B, Stone NJ, et al. Relation of body mass index to late survival after valvular heart surgery. Am J Cardiol. 2012 Dec;110(11):1667-78.

51. Huang PL. A comprehensive definition for metabolic syndrome. Dis Model Mech. 2009 May;2(5-6):231-7.

52. Mathieu P. Abdominal obesity and the metabolic syndrome: a surgeon's perspective. Can J Cardiol. 2008 Sep;24 Suppl 4:19-23.

53. Briand M, Pibarot P, Despres JP, Voisine P, Dumesnil JG, Dagenais F, et al. Metabolic syndrome is associated with faster degeneration of bioprosthetic valves. Circulation. 2006 Jul;114 Suppl 1:512-7.

54. Haute Autorite de Sante. Guide du parcours de soins - Maladie renale chronique de I'adulte (MRC) [On line]. Oct 2023 [Accessed 24 Sep 2023]. Available at URL: https://www.has-sante.fr/jcms/p_3288950/fr/guide-du-parcours-de-soins-maladie-   renale-chronique-de-l'-adulte-mrc

55. Schoen FJ, Golomb G, Levy RJ. Calcification of bioprosthetic heart valves: a perspective on models. J Heart Valve Dis. 1992 Sep;1(1):110-4.

56. Zhibing Q, Xin C, Ming X, Lele L, YingSJ, LiMW. Should bioprostheses be considered the

valve of choice for dialysis-dependent patients? J Cardiothorac Surg. 2013 Mar;8:42.

57. Kumar RK, Tandon R. Rheumatic fever & rheumatic heart disease: the last 50 years. Indian J Med Res. 2013 Apr;137(4):643-58.

58. Nashef SM, Roques F, Sharples LD, Nilsson J, Smith C, Goldstone AR, et al. EuroSCORE II. Eur J Cardiothorac Surg. 2012 Apr;41(4):734-44.

59. Casalino R, Tarasoutchi F, Spina G, Katz M, Bacelar A, Sampaio R, et al. EuroSCORE models in a cohort of patients with valvular heart disease and a high prevalence of rheumatic fever submitted to surgical procedures. PLoS One. 2015 Feb;10(2):e0118357.

60. Czub P, Cacko A, Gawalko M, Tataj E, Polinski J, Pawlik K, et al. Perioperative risk assessment with Euroscore and Euroscore II in patients with coronary artery or valvular disease. Medicine. 2018 Dec;97(50):e13572.

61. Boudoulas H. Etiology of valvular heart disease. Expert Rev Cardiovasc Ther. 2003 Nov;1(4):523-32.

62. Habib G, Lancellotti P, Antunes MJ, Bongiorni MG, Casalta JP, Del Zotti F, et al. 2015 ESC guidelines for the management of infective endocarditis: the task force for the management of infective endocarditis of the European society of cardiology (ESC). Endorsed by: European Association for cardio-thoracic surgery (EACTS), the European association of nuclear medicine (EANM). Eur Heart J. 2015 Nov;36(44):3075-128.

63. Hoffman JIE, Kaplan S. The incidence of congenital heart disease. J Am Coll Cardiol. 2002 Jun;39(12):1890-900.

64. Verma R, Cohen G, Colbert J, Fedak PM. Bicuspid aortic valve associated aortopathy: 2022 guideline update. Curr Opin Cardiol. 2023 Mar;38(2):61-7.

65. Melnitchouk SI, Seeburger J, Kaeding AF, Misfeld M, Mohr FW, Borger MA. Barlow's mitral valve disease: results of conventional and minimally invasive repair approaches. Ann Cardiothorac Surg. 2013 Nov;2(6):768-73.

66. Park SJ, Enriquez Sarano M, Chang SA, Choi JO, Lee SC, Park SW, et al. Hemodynamic patterns for symptomatic presentations of severe aortic stenosis. JACC Cardiovasc Imaging. 2013 Feb;6(2):137-46.

67. Goliasch G, Kammerlander AA, Nitsche C, Dona C, Schachner L, Ozturk B, et al. Syncope: the underestimated threat in severe aortic stenosis. JACC Cardiovasc Imaging. 2019 Feb;12(2):225-32.

68. Fan Y, Pui Wai Lee A. Valvular disease and heart failure with preserved ejection fraction. Heart Fail Clin. 2021 Jul;17(3):387-95.

69. Messe SR, Acker MA, Kasner SE, Fanning M, Giovannetti T, Ratcliffe SJ, et al. Stroke after aortic valve surgery. Circulation. 2014 Jun;129(22):2253-61.

70. Chua YL, Schaff HV, Orszulak TA, Morris JJ. Outcome of mitral valve repair in patients with preoperative atrial fibrillation: should the maze procedure be combined with mitral valvuloplasty? J Thorac Cardiovasc Surg. 1994 Feb;107(2):408-15.

71. Haq IU, Haq I, Griffin B, Xu B. Imaging to evaluate suspected infective endocarditis. Cleve Clin J Med. 2021 Mar;88(3):163-72.

72. Chen JJ, Manning MA, Frazier AA, Jeudy J, White CS. CT angiography of the cardiac valves: normal, diseased, and postoperative appearances. Radiographics. 2009 Sep;29(5):1393-412.

73. Chenot F, Montant P, Goffinet C, Pasquet A, Vancraeynest D, Coche E, et al. Evaluation of anatomic valve opening and leaflet morphology in aortic valve bioprosthesis by using multidetector CT: comparison with transthoracic echocardiography. Radiology. 2010 May;255(2):377-85.

74. Muthialu N, Varma SK, Ramanathan S, Padmanabhan C, Rao KM, Srinivasan M. Effect of chordal preservation on left ventricular function. Asian Cardiovasc Thorac Ann. 2005 Sep;13(3):233-7.

75. Anselmi A, Ruggieri VG, Harmouche M, Flecher E, Corbineau H, Langanay T, et al. Appraisal of long-term outcomes of tricuspid valve replacement in the current perspective. Ann Thorac Surg. 2016 Mar;101(3):863-71.

76. Elmistekawy E, Mesana TG. Tricuspid valve operations. In: Sellke FW, Ruel M, eds Atlas of cardiac surgical techniques (second edition). Paris: Elsevier; 2019. p. 384-406.

77. Puvimanasinghe JA, Takkenberg JM, Eijkemans MC, Steyerberg EW, Van Herwerden LA, Grunkemeier GL, et al. Choice of a mechanical valve or a bioprosthesis for AVR: does CABG matter? Eur J Cardiothorac Surg. 2003 May;23(5):688-95.

78. De Freitas Campos Guimaraes L, Urena M, Wijeysundera HC, Munoz Garcia A, Serra V, Benitez LM, et al. Long-term outcomes after transcatheter aortic valve-in-valve replacement. Circ Cardiovasc Interv. 2018 Sep;11(9):e007038.

79. Ibrahim KS, Kheirallah KA, Mayyas FA, Alwaqfi NR, Alawami MH, Aljarrah QM. Predictors of short-term mortality after rheumatic heart valve surgery: a single-center retrospective study. Ann Med Surg. 2021 Jan;62:395-401.

80. Landes U, Sathananthan J, Witberg G, De Backer O, Sondergaard L, Abdel Wahab M, et al. Transcatheter replacement of transcatheter versus surgically implanted aortic valve bioprostheses. J Am Coll Cardiol. 2021 Jan;77(1):1-14.

81. Ferreira R, Rua N, Sena A, Velho TR, Goncalves J, Junqueira N, et al. Sutureless bioprosthesis for aortic valve replacement: surgical and clinical outcomes. J Card Surg. 2022 Dec;37(12):4774-82.

82. Ramsaransing K, Hindori V, Kougioumtzoglou A, Kaya A, Verbeek E. Minimally invasive sutureless aortic valve replacement with the perceval S bioprosthesis through ministernotomy: a single-center experience. Cureus. 2020 Oct;12(10):e11212.

83. Shrestha M, Maeding I, Hoffler K, Koigeldiyev N, Marsch G, Siemeni T, et al. Aortic valve replacement in geriatric patients with small aortic roots: are sutureless valves the future? Interact Cardiovasc Thorac Surg. 2013 Nov;17(5):778-82.

84. Guner Y, Qi^ek A, Karacalilar M, Ersoy B, Kyaruzi M, Onan B. Comparison of postoperative outcomes of sutureless versus stented bioprosthetic aortic valve replacement. Braz J Cardiovasc Surg. 2022 May;37(3):328-34.

85. Fang ZA, Navaei AH, Hensch L, Hui SR, Teruya J. Hemostatic management of extracorporeal circuits including cardiopulmonary bypass and extracorporeal membrane oxygenation. Semin Thromb Hemost. 2020 Feb;46(1):62-72.

86. Kristensen KL, Rauer LJ, Mortensen PE, Kjeldsen BJ. Reoperation for bleeding in cardiac surgery. Interact Cardiovasc Thorac Surg. 2012 Jun;14(6):709-13.

87. Canadyova J, Zmeko D, Mokracek A. Re-exploration for bleeding or tamponade after cardiac operation. Interact Cardiovasc Thorac Surg. 2012 Jun;14(6):704-7.

88. Kuvin JT, Harati NA, Pandian NG, Bojar RM, Khabbaz KR. Postoperative cardiac tamponade in the modern surgical era. Ann Thorac Surg. 2002 Oct;74(4):1148-53.

89. Uzun K, Gunaydin ZY, Tataroglu C, Bekta§ O. The preventive role of the posterior pericardial window in the development of late cardiac tamponade following heart valve surgery. Interact Cardiovasc Thorac Surg. 2016 May;22(5):641-6.

90. Lagier D, Fischer F, Fornier W, Huynh TM, Cholley B, Guinard B, et al. Effect of openlung vs conventional perioperative ventilation strategies on postoperative pulmonary complications after on-pump cardiac surgery: the PROVECS randomized clinical trial.

Intensive Care Med. 2019 Oct;45(10):1401-12.

91. Kollef MH, Sharpless L, Vlasnik J, Pasque C, Murphy D, Fraser VJ. The impact of nosocomial infections on patient outcomes following cardiac surgery. Chest. 1997 Sep;112(3):666-75.

92. Xiao P, Song W, Han Z. Characteristics of pulmonary infection after mitral valve repair in patients with metabolic syndrome and its relationship with blood pressure, blood glucose and blood lipid. Exp Ther Med. 2018 Dec;16(6):5003-8.

93. Riera M, Ibanez J, Herrero J, De Ibarra J, Ennquez F, Campillo C, et al. Respiratory tract infections after cardiac surgery: impact on hospital morbidity and mortality. J Cardiovasc Surg. 2010 Dec;51(6):907-14.

94. Filardo G, Hamilton C, Hamman B, Hebeler RF, Adams J, Grayburn P. New-onset postoperative atrial fibrillation and long-term survival after aortic valve replacement surgery. Ann Thorac Surg. 2010 Aug;90(2):474-9.

95. Kalra R, Patel N, Doshi R, Arora G, Arora P. Evaluation of the incidence of new-onset atrial fibrillation after aortic valve replacement. JAMA Intern Med. 2019 Aug;179(8):1122-30.

96. Bjorn R, Nissinen M, Lehto J, Malmberg M, Yannopoulos F, Airaksinen KJ, et al. Late incidence and recurrence of new-onset atrial fibrillation after isolated surgical aortic valve replacement. J Thorac Cardiovasc Surg. 2022 Dec;164(6):1833-43.

97. Merin O, Ilan M, Oren A, Fink D, Deeb M, Bitran D, et al. Permanent pacemaker implantation following cardiac surgery: indications and long-term follow-up. Pacing Clin Electrophysiol. 2009 Jan;32(1):7-12.

98. Ferrari ADL, Sussenbach CP, Guaragna JC, Piccoli JE, Gazzoni GF, Ferreira DK, et al. Bloqueio atrioventricular no pos-operatorio de cirurgia cardi'aca valvar: incidence, risk factors and hospital evolution. Rev Bras Cir Cardiovasc. 2011 Jul;26(3):364-72.

99. Viles Gonzalez JF, Enriquez AD, Castillo JG, Coffey JO, Pastori L, Reddy VY, et al. Incidence, predictors, and evolution of conduction disorders and atrial arrhythmias after contemporary mitral valve repair. Cardiol J. 2014;21(5):569-75.

100. Elahi M, Usmaan K. The bioprosthesis type and size influence the postoperative incidence of permanent pacemaker implantation in patients undergoing aortic valve surgery. J Interv Card Electrophysiol. 2006 Mar;15(2):113-8.

101. Gaudino M, Dangas GD, Angiolillo DJ, Brodt J, Chikwe J, DeAnda A, et al. Considerations on the management of acute postoperative ischemia after cardiac surgery: a scientific statement from the American heart association. Circulation. 2023 Aug;148(5):442-54.

102. Wang A, Fosb0l EL. Current recommendations and uncertainties for surgical treatment of infective endocarditis: a comparison of American and European cardiovascular guidelines. Eur Heart J. 2022 May;43(17):1617-25.

103. Nagpal A, Sohail MR, Steckelberg JM. Prosthetic valve endocarditis: state of the heart. J Clin Invest. 2012 Jul;2(8):803-17.

104. Stassano P, Di Tommaso L, Monaco M, Iorio F, Pepino P, Spampinato N, et al. Aortic valve replacement: a prospective randomized evaluation of mechanical versus biological valves in patients ages 55 to 70 years. J Am Coll Cardiol. 2009 Nov;54(20):1862-8.

105. Egbe AC, Connolly HM, Pellikka PA, Schaff HV, Hanna R, Maleszewski JJ, et al. Outcomes of warfarin therapy for bioprosthetic valve thrombosis of surgically implanted valves: a prospective study. JACC Cardiovasc Interv. 2017 Feb;10(4):379-87.

106. Oliver JM, Gallego P, Gonzalez A, Dominguez FJ, Gamallo C, Mesa JM. Bioprosthetic mitral valve thrombosis: clinical profile, transesophageal echocardiographic features, and

follow-up after anticoagulant therapy. J Am Soc Echocardiogr. 1996 Sep;9(5):691-9.

107.   Dvir D, Bourguignon T, Otto CM, Hahn RT, Rosenhek R, Webb JG, et al. Standardized definition of structural valve degeneration for surgical and transcatheter bioprosthetic aortic valves. Circulation. 2018 Jan;137(4):388-99.

108.   Cote N, Pibarot P, Clavel MA. Incidence, risk factors, clinical impact, and management of bioprosthesis structural valve degeneration. Curr Opin Cardiol. 2017 Mar;32(2):123-29.

109.   Belluschi I, Buzzatti N, Castiglioni A, De Bonis M, Maisano F, Alfieri O. Aortic and mitral bioprosthetic valve dysfunction: surgical or percutaneous solutions? Eur Heart J Suppl. 2021 Oct;23 Suppl 2:6-12.

110.   Guenzinger R, Fiegl K, Wottke M, Lange RS. Twenty-seven-year experience with the St. Jude medical biocor bioprosthesis in the aortic position. Ann Thorac Surg. 2015 Dec;100(6):2220-6.

111.   Neville PH, Aupart MR, Diemont FF, Sirinelli AL, Lemoine EM, Marchand MA. Carpentier- Edwards pericardial bioprosthesis in aortic or mitral position: a 12-year experience. Ann Thorac Surg. 1998 Dec;66 Suppl 6:S143-7.

112.   Raghav V, Okafor I, Quach M, Dang L, Marquez S, Yoganathan AP. Long-term durability of carpentier-edwards magna ease valve: a one billion cycle in vitro study. Ann Thorac Surg. 2016 May;101(5):1759-65.

113.   Ruiz CE, Jelnin V, Kronzon I, Dudiy Y, Del ValleFernandez R, Einhorn BN, et al. Clinical outcomes in patients undergoing percutaneous closure of periprosthetic paravalvular leaks. J Am Coll Cardiol. 2011 Nov;58(21):2210-7.

114.   W^sowicz M, Meineri M, Djaiani G, Mitsakakis N, Hegazi N, Xu W, et al. Early complications and immediate postoperative outcomes of paravalvular leaks after valve replacement surgery. J Cardiothorac Vasc Anesth. 2011 Aug;25(4):610-4.

115.   Allen KB, Chhatriwalla AK, Saxon JT, Huded CP, Sathananthan J, Nguyen TC, et al. Bioprosthetic valve fracture: a practical guide. Ann Cardiothorac Surg. 2021 Sep;10(5):564-70.

116.   Asimakopoulos G, Edwards MB, Taylor KM. Aortic valve replacement in patients 80 years of age and older. Circulation. 1997 Nov;96(10):3403-8.

117.   Suri RM, Thourani VH, Englum BR, Rankin JS, Badhwar V, Svensson LG, et al. The expanding role of mitral valve repair in triple valve operations: contemporary north American outcomes in 8,021 patients. Ann Thorac Surg. 2014 May;97(5):1513-9.

Appendix 1: Data collection form

- File number :
- Patient's full name :
- Phone number :
- Service of origin :
- Gender: 0. male 1. Female
- Age: Weight: Height: BMI :

Treatment in progress :

- Aspegic: 0.yes 1.no
- Insulin: 0.yes 1.no

Medical history:

- Rheumatic fever: 0.yes l.no
- Diabetes: Y.yes l.no
- Tobacco: Y.yes l.no
- HTA: Y.yes l.no
- Dyslipidemia: Y.yes l.no
- Coronary artery disease: O.yes l.no If yes: Medical: O.yes l.no Stent O.yes l.no
- Endocarditis: Y.yes l.no
- COPD O.yes l.no
- Stroke O.yes l.no
- Chronic renal failure : Y.yes l.no, Creat : Hemodialysis : Y.yes l.no

Previous surgery :

- Cardiac surgery: Y.yes l.no if yes Bypass surgery: Y.yes l.no
- Rvao : Y.yes l.no
- RVM: Y.yes l.no
- CMCF: Y.yes l.no

Euroscore :

Emergency context: Y.yes l.no

Response times :

Etiologies :

- Rheumatic: Y.yes l.no
- Degenerative: Y.yes l.no
- Endocarditis: Y.yes l.no
- Libman-sacks : Y.yes l.no
- Bicuspidity: Y.yes l.no
- Hypertensive heart disease: Y.yes l.no
- Barlow's disease: Y.yes l.no

Clinical data :

- Dyspnea: Y.yes l.no if yes NYHA :
- Right heart failure: Y.yes l.no
- Left heart failure: Y.yes l.no
- Syncope and equivalent: Y.yes l.no
- Chest pain: Y.yes l.no
- Embolic: Y.yes l.no

Paraclinical data :
Chest X-ray :
- Cardiomegaly: Y.yes I.no
- Coil overload: Y.yes I.no
- Double contour: Y.yes I.no

ECG :
- FA: Y.yes I.no
- Conduction disorder: Y.yes I.no
- Repolarisation disorder: Y.yes I.no

Coronary angiography :
- Significant lesion: Y.yes I.no
- Intervention (associated bypass): Y.yes I.no

ETSA :
Significant lesion: Y.yes I.no

Echocardiography :
- FE: PAPS :
- HVG: Y.yes I.no
- LV dilation: Y.yes I.no
- VD dilation: Y.yes I.no
- Aortic valve: Y.yes I.no if yes Aortic surface :
- Aortic narrowing: Y.yes I.no Mean gradient :
- Aortic insufficiency: Y.yes I.no
- Mitral valve: Y.yes I.no
- If yes Mitral narrowing: Y.yes I.no Mitral surface :
- Average gradient :
- Mitral insufficiency: Y.yes I.no
- Prolapse: Y.yes I.no
- Tricuspid insufficiency: Y.yes I.no

Associated valve lesions:
- Vegetation : Y.yes I.no
- Abces : 0.yes 1.no
- Thrombus: 0.yes 1.no

Intraoperative management :
- Clamping time :
- CEC time :
- Catecholamines: Without catecholamines: Y.yes I.no
- Low dose: Y.yes I.no
- High dose: Y.yes I.no
- Approach: Vertical median sternotomy: Y.yes I.no Mini-sternotomy: Y.yes I.no

Actions taken :
- Mitral valve replacement: Y.yes I.no Size: Brand :
- Aortic valve replacement: Y.yes I.no Size: Brand :
- Tricuspid gesture: Replacement: Y.yes I.no Annuloplasty: Y.yes I.no Size: Make :
- Death on table: Y.yes I.no

Resuscitation :
- Length of stay in intensive care :
- Intubation time :

- Antibiotics: Y.yes I.no
- Anticoagualtion: Curative: Y.yes I.no Preventive: Y.yes I.no

Cardiac complications :

- ACFA : Y.yes I.no BAV : Y.yes I.no Pace : Y.yes I.no Hypertensive peak : Y.yes I.no
- Infective endocarditis: Y.yes I.no Valve thrombosis: Y.yes I.no MI: Y.yes I.no
- Tamponnade: Y.yes I.no

Pulmonary complications :

- Infection: Y.yes I.no
- Acute lung disease: Y.yes I.no

Other complications:

- Postoperative bleeding: Y.yes I.no Recovery: Y.yes I.no
- Cerebrovascular accident: Y.yes I.no
- Mediastinitis: 0.yes I.no
- Length of stay :

Remote results :

Clinical :

- Dyspnea: Y.yes I.no
- Heart failure: Y.yes I.no
- Syncope: Y.yes I.no
- Chest pain: Y.yes I.no

ECG :

- FA : Y.yes I.no
- BAV: Y.yes I.no Pace-maker: Y.yes I.no
- Repolarisation disorder: Y.yes I.no

Post-operative ultrasound :

- Ultrasound control: Y.yes I.no EF: PAPS: LVH: Y.yes I.no
- Dilatation of the VD: Y.yes I.no
- Intracavitary thrombus: Y.yes I.no
- Valve profile preserved : O.yes I.no
- Leaky prosthesis : O.yes I.no
- Stenosing prosthesis : Y.yes I.no

Mortality :

- Death on operating table: Y.yes I.no
- Death within 30 days: Y.yes I.no
- Death at one year: Y.yes I.no

Appendix 2: EACTS recommendations for the choice of valve prosthesis :

Recommendations	Class[a]	Level[b]
Mechanical prostheses		
A mechanical prosthesis is recommended according to the desire of the informed patient and if there are no contraindications to long-term anticoagulation.[c]	I	C
A mechanical prosthesis is recommended in patients at risk of accelerated SVD.[d]	I	C
A mechanical prosthesis should be considered in patients already on anticoagulation because of a mechanical prosthesis in another valve position.	IIa	C
A mechanical prosthesis should be considered in patients aged <60 years for prostheses in the aortic position and aged <65 years for prostheses in the mitral position.[162, 464 e]	IIa	B
A mechanical prosthesis should be considered in patients with a reasonable life expectancy for whom future redo valve surgery or TAVI (if appropriate) would be at high risk.[f]	IIa	C
A mechanical prosthesis may be considered in patients already on long-term anticoagulation due to the high risk for thromboembolism.[f]	IIb	C

Biological prostheses		
A bioprosthesis is recommended according to the desire of the informed patient.	I	C
A bioprosthesis is recommended when good-quality anticoagulation is unlikely (adherence problems, not readily available), contraindicated because of high bleeding risk (previous major bleed, comorbidities, unwillingness, adherence problems, lifestyle, occupation) and in those patients whose life expectancy is lower than the presumed durability of the bioprosthesis.[g]	I	C
A bioprosthesis is recommended in case of reoperation for mechanical valve thrombosis despite good long-term anticoagulant control.	I	C
A bioprosthesis should be considered in patients for whom there is a low likelihood and/or a low operative risk of future redo valve surgery.	IIa	C
A bioprosthesis should be considered in young women contemplating pregnancy.	IIa	C
A bioprosthesis should be considered in patients aged >65 years for a prosthesis in the aortic position or aged >70 years in a mitral position.	IIa	C
A bioprosthesis may be considered in patients already on long-term NOACs due to the high risk for thromboembolism.[166–169 f]	IIb	B

Medium- and long-term results of valve bioprostheses: A Tunisian multicentric study

Abstract

Introduction:

The use of cardiacbioprostheses is steadily increasing. Thanks to their haemodynamic characteristics, longevity and the fact that they do not require anticoagulant treatment, bioprostheses have become the alternative of choice for patients of all ages.

The aim of the study is to analyze the profile of patients who have undergone valve replacement by bioprosthesis, and study the factors predictive of morbidity and mortality.

Materials and Methods:

This is a retrospective, multicentric, descriptive, cross-sectional study conducted in the cardiovascular surgery departments of the AbderrahmenMami University Hospital in Ariana, the Habib Bourguiba University Hospital in Sfax, and the Tunis Military Hospital, between September 2017 and December 2021.

Results:

This study included 106 patients undergoing valve replacement with a bioprosthesis in any position. The mean age of the patients included in the study was 68 years, with an estimated age range of 9% between 17 and 45 years.

23 patients required emergency surgery (21.7%) following a complication. Six intraoperative deaths were reported.

We noted 54% of infectious pneumopathies, 24% of postoperative bleeding, 16 of which were required re-intervention, 17% of acute pulmonary oedema, 11% of postoperative tamponade, and 9% of mediastinitis. Only one case of early intermittent obstructive thrombosis of a mitral prosthesis was reported.

During the post-operative period, 21 early deaths occurred, giving an in-hospital mortality rate of 25.4%. Only one late death was reported, of undetermined cause.

The mean follow-up was 54.5 months. Follow-up echocardiography revealed a good haemodynamic profile for the bioprostheses implanted in 90.9% of cases, a stenosing bioprosthesis in 4 patients (6%) and two leaking prostheses (3%).

We identified the following factors as predictive of mortality: overweight, aortic valve insufficiency, administration of catecholamines, emergency valve surgery, prolonged operation time and postoperative pulmonary infections.

Conclusion:

Bioprostheses offer a satisfying quality of life with promising results in terms of sustainability and functionality. However, further work is still needed to study the long-term evolution in the young population.

Keywords: heart surgery, extracorporeal circulation, bioprosthesis, aortic valve, mitral valve, heart valve prosthesis implantation. [125]

Resume

Introduction :

The use of cardiac bioprostheses is constantly increasing. Thanks to their hemodynamic characteristics, their longevity and the fact that they do not require anticoagulant treatment, bioprostheses have become the alternative of choice for patients of all ages.

The aim of this study is to describe the profile of patients who have undergone bioprosthetic valve replacement, and to investigate the factors predictive of morbidity and mortality.

Materials and methods :

This is a retrospective, multicentre, descriptive, cross-sectional study conducted in the cardiovascular surgery departments of the Abderrahmen-Mami University Hospital in Ariana, the Habib Bourguiba University Hospital in Sfax, and the Tunis Military Hospital, between September 2017 and December 2021.

Results:

This study included 106 patients undergoing valve replacement with a bioprosthesis in any position. The mean age of the patients included in the study was 68 years, with an estimated 9% aged between 17 and 45 years.

23 patients required emergency surgery (21.7%) following a complication. Six per-operative deaths were reported.

We noted 54% of infectious pneumopathies, 24% of post-operative bleeding, of which 16 were repaired, 17% of acute lung re-infarction, 11% of post-operative tamponade, and 9% of mediastinitis. Only one early intermittent obstructive thrombosis of a mitral prosthesis was reported.

During the post-operative period, 21 early deaths occurred, giving a hospital mortality rate of 25.4%. Only one late death was reported without a cause.

The mean follow-up was 54.5 months. Follow-up echocardiography revealed a good hemodynamic profile for the bioprostheses implanted in 90.9% of cases, a stenosing bioprosthesis in 4 patients (6%) and two leaky prostheses (3%).

We identified the following factors as predictive of mortality: overweight, leaky aortic valve disease, administration of catecholamines, valve surgery performed in an emergency setting, prolonged operating times and post-operative pulmonary infections.

Conclusion:

Bioprostheses offer a satisfactory quality of life, with promising results in terms of durability and functionality. However, further work is still needed to study the long-term evolution in the young population.

Key words : Cardiac surgery - Extracorporeal circulation - Bioprosthesis - Aortic valve - Mitral valve - Heart valve replacement.

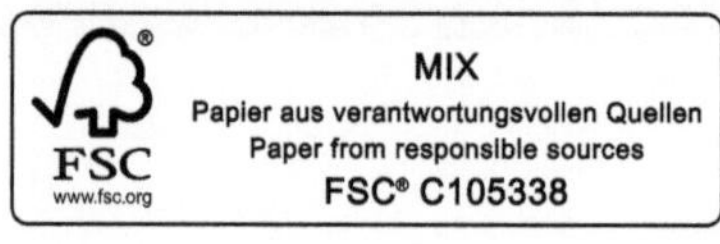

Printed by Books on Demand GmbH, Norderstedt / Germany